Child and Infant Pain

Child and Infant Pain

PRINCIPLES OF NURSING CARE
AND MANAGEMENT

Bernadette Carter

Senior Lecturer in Health Care Studies
the Manchester Metropolitan University
Manchester, UK

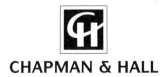

CHAPMAN & HALL

London · Glasgow · Weinheim · New York · Tokyo · Melbourne · Madras

Published by Chapman & Hall, 2–6 Boundary Row, London SE1 8HN, UK

Chapman & Hall, 2–6 Boundary Row, London SE1 8HN, UK

Blackie Academic & Professional, Wester Cleddens Road, Bishopbriggs, Glasgow G64 2NZ, UK

Chapman & Hall GmbH, Pappelallee 3, 69469 Weinheim, Germany

Chapman & Hall USA, One Penn Plaza, 41st Floor, New York NY 10119, USA

Chapman & Hall Japan, ITP-Japan, Kyowa Building, 3F, 2-2-1 Hirakawacho, Chiyoda-ku, Tokyo 102, Japan

Chapman & Hall Australia, Thomas Nelson Australia, 102 Dodds Street, South Melbourne, Victoria 3205, Australia

Chapman & Hall India, R. Seshadri, 32 Second Main Road, CIT East, Madras 600 035, India

Distributed in the USA and Canada by Singular Publishing Group Inc., 4284 41st Street, San Diego, California 92105

First edition 1994

© 1994 Chapman & Hall

Typeset in 10/12 Times by Mews Photosetting, Beckenham, Kent
Printed in Great Britain by St Edmundsbury Press, Bury St Edmunds, Suffolk

ISBN 0 412 48720 9   1 56593 181 5 (USA)

A catalogue record for this book is available from the British Library

Library of Congress Catalog Card Number: 94-71198

♾ Printed on permanent acid-free text paper, manufactured in accordance with the proposed ANSI/NISO Z39.48-1992 and ANSI/NISO Z39.48-1984 (Permanence of Paper).

For Angela and Louise;
and Jon.

'Pain is a critical ethical issue
because of its capacity to
dehumanize the human person'
(Lisson, 1987)

Contents

Preface

This book intends to act as a resource for those caring for children. The children I nursed who experienced pain are the stimulus for both my interest in the issue of pain and latterly in writing this book. Some of the children I cared for stand out as milestones in terms of provoking thought and in questioning practice – James, Ralph and Felicity. These children were tough and brave and taught me a lot about the human aspect of pain and suffering. However, as children, especially vulnerable children in hospital, they would not have had to have been as tough or as brave if I had been more knowledgeable about practice issues such as distraction, imagery, massage and so on or had a better understanding of the complexity of pain.

Nursing should add to a child's life. By developing knowledge and skills within pain management and prevention nurses are in a strong position to ensure that they, the child and their family are in control of the pain and that the pain is not in control of the child. Developing these skills is ultimately rewarding both personally and professionally and nurses should be encouraged to scrutinize their practice carefully and identify areas where improvements could be made. Listening carefully to what children and their families say about their pain and in identifying the needs of the individual child is an essential part of holistic and comprehensive nursing care. Whilst researching this book I took the opportunity to interview children and their families during their admission to hospital. Again the complexity of pain was obvious both in terms of the effects it had on the children (physically and psychologically) and to some degree what they wanted their nurses to do. The additional insight I gained from letting them tell me their stories was vital. Overwhelmingly the children wanted to have someone with them if they were in pain and they were all relatively sophisticated in the way in which they were able to describe their experiences and their needs. I am deeply grateful for the time that the children and their families gave me when I was interviewing them. I am also grateful for the support and help given me by the staff at the Royal Hospital for Sick Children, Pendlebury, Manchester, who continue to be strongly committed and motivated in respect to pain management.

Bernie Carter

Pain in perspective | 1

INTRODUCTION

Children and infants, like the rest of humanity, can and do perceive and experience pain. Many misconceptions have, until relatively recently, been held by health professionals about children's and infants' ability to perceive and experience pain. Of all of these perhaps the most fundamentally damaging one was the myth that children and infants were unable to perceive and experience pain. This myth, which has now been rejected, has allowed and perhaps even encouraged the dismissal of pain as an issue, and chronic mismanagement of the child in pain has resulted. Thankfully pain is now an issue that the nurse and the rest of the multidisciplinary team cannot ignore. Pain is now accepted as an area of fundamental responsibility for the nurse which is important; however, what is more important is that responsibility is fulfilled with all children and their families. Effective pain management starts with a commitment to believe in the pain that the child is reporting and to work with them and their family to achieve the best level of control that is possible. Pain management is based on honesty and trust and effective communication skills; without these essential skills pain management will be flawed.

Children and infants have a right to careful consideration and management of their pain and it is the duty of every nurse to ensure that this right is fulfilled. Children may experience pain in a different way from adults but this does not mean to say that their experience is of less importance than adult experiences. Indeed when considering their vulnerability and lack of autonomy it achieves a special importance. Children need effective pain management to ensure that their experience of illness or injury is as atraumatic as possible. Nurses must develop their skills and deepen their knowledge on pain and pain management to ensure that they provide high-quality care.

Pain is a problem in its own right. Children's experience of pain is often separate from their experience of the illness or disease that care givers may associate the pain with. Despite the increased attention that pain management has received it is unfortunate that a proportion of children receiving care do not receive adequate care in respect of their pain. This must be addressed and nurses should make stringent efforts to ensure that they and their colleagues develop a firm commitment to pain management. As with adults, children have different experiences and reactions to pain from the same stimulus, and the relationship between the pain stimulus and the response is not direct or simple. This provides a challenge that nurses must respond to and meet.

DEFINING PAIN

Many words have been written defining pain and they provide a framework upon which to build assessment and evaluation tools – a common base from which to confer with colleagues and a baseline for research. However, the definitions themselves rarely convey the quality of the experience of pain. Defining pain is difficult: it is a complicated and elusive concept for someone outside of the experience to convey in words. Dictionary definitions are not much help as they explain the word but not the experience. For example:

> [Pain is] the sensation of acute physical hurt or discomfort caused by injury, illness, etc. . . . emotional suffering or mental distress.
>
> (*Collins English Dictionary*, 1991)

The word pain is derived from the Latin word *poena*, which means punishment, which is in turn derived from the Sanscrit root *pu*, meaning purification. In many languages the word has its derivation associated with suffering, punishment and anxiety although this is not exclusively the case. In languages such as Russian, German and Hebrew there is no punitive association with the word equivalent to pain. Ultimately these meanings associated with words for pain are strongly reflective of the specific cultural attitudes towards the phenomenon of pain. Pain within Western culture is often seen as being synonymous with wrongdoing and punishment and this often makes pain harder to bear, especially for the child.

Many definitions have been proposed although none of them perhaps completely defines the experience that pain presents. Sternbach (1968) proposed that:

> pain is an abstract concept which refers to:
>
> 1. a personal, private sensation of hurt;
> 2. a harmful stimulus which signifies current or impending tissue damage;
> 3. a pattern of impulses which operate to protect the organism from harm.

However, the definition that holds the widest credence and is used the most consistently is the official International Association for the Study of Pain definition which was published in 1979:

an unpleasant sensory and emotional experience with actual or potential tissue damage, or described in terms of such damage. Pain is always
subjective. Each individual learns the application of the word through
experiences related to injury in early life.

This definition is useful inasmuch as it acknowledges the subjectivity, emotional and sensory nature of the experience. It also acknowledges that early
experience during childhood provides the basis for understanding the 'meaning' of the word pain. This aspect is of crucial importance to children's nurses
who may be able to help to reduce the trauma associated with the word pain.
   McCaffery (1979) attempts to define pain by using a patient-centred
approach and her definition is now widely accepted and frequently quoted,
even if it is not always acted upon:

   pain is whatever the experiencing person says it is, existing whenever
   he says it does.

The difficulty of this definition in respect to children and especially infants
is that often the child is unable to locate, define and describe 'it'. Difficulty
in verbalizing pain experiences has made it easier for nurses and doctors to
ignore the issue as the child's pain cues can be misinterpreted. However, it
is part of the nurses' responsibility to the children in their care to develop
the skill of interpreting the range of signals and the information that children
give. Perhaps the most obvious person to ask about a definition of pain is
the child – alas this is something which is not done very frequently. However,
when interviewing one 7-year-old boy and asking if he could tell me what
he thought pain was he looked me straight in the eye and sighed heavily and
then said:

   Pain hurts – stupid!

                                             (Jonathan, aged 7 years)

This perhaps sums up pain fairly succintly and reminded me that 7-year-olds
do not tolerate what they perceive to be daft questions.
   Children can often communicate something of the quality of their pain
experience by the use of drawings which can be very powerful ways of
demonstrating the impact that pain has had on their lives. Both physical and
emotional pain can be potently illustrated as can be seen in Figs 1.1 and 1.2.
   'Suffering' and 'unpleasant experience' although accurate semantically does
little to describe the intensity of an experience or of the effects that the
experience may have on the child. The definitions themselves often reflect
the background of the person or group and this must be borne in mind before
accepting the definition. The usefulness of the definition should also be
considered.
   Pain is a unique and complicated experience for children and infants – unique
not only to the child experiencing it but also unique to all other experiences

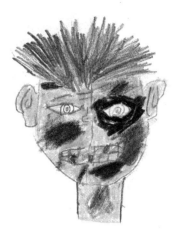

Figure 1.1 Stuart has undergone repeated surgery and has experienced many invasive procedures.

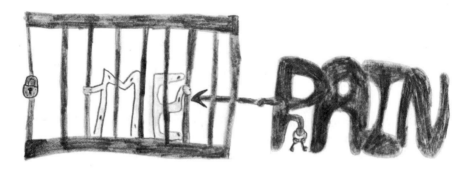

Figure 1.2 Kathryn illustrates her experience of both emotional and physical pain.

of pain that that child has had. Pain is often an all-consuming experience for a child and one which they often find difficulty in explaining to adults. This is not surprising considering the difficulties faced in trying to define the concept of pain itself.

TYPES AND EFFECTS OF PAIN

Pain is often defined in terms of duration: acute pain and chronic pain with further subdivisions within the chronic category. However, the boundaries between the two categories are not always clear and pain may also be categorized according to the presumed origin: nociceptive (tissue damage); neuropathic (nerve damage); and psychogenic (predominantly psychological) (Justins, 1991).

Acute pain is usually characterized by its relatively brief duration (less than six months); it subsides as healing occurs although a child experiencing brief pain is unlikely to perceive its duration as being brief. It is the most common pain experienced by infants and children. They generally experience acute pain as a result of the injuries and accidents that are a normal part of growing up or as a result of invasive painful procedures such as those experienced at the dentist and the doctor's or the hospital. However, acute pain does resolve. McCaffery and Beebe (1989) state about acute pain that it:

> also may be either sudden or slow in onset and may be of any intensity; ranging from mild to severe. (p. 19)

Chronic pain/chronic persistent pain is prolonged and is generally agreed to last three months or longer (Schechter *et al.*, 1993) or more than six months (McCaffery and Beebe, 1989). The International Association for the Study of Pain defines chronic pain as pain persisting past the normal time of healing, most commonly approximately three months. Implicit in this definition is that factors apart from nociception due to injury are probably involved (Merskey, 1986). McCaffery and Beebe (1989) further subdivide prolonged pain into: recurrent acute pain; ongoing time-limited or chronic acute; and chronic non-malignant or chronic benign pain.

Recurrent acute pain occurs over a prolonged period or even a lifetime. The pain episodes are self-contained and predictable and the child is pain free between episodes such as in migraine headaches, sickle cell crises and abdominal pains. McGrath (1990) reports that 'approximately 30% of children and adolescents may experience recurrent headaches or abdominal pains' (p. 14). There is evidence to suggest that children who experience this type of pain over a long period of time are at increased risk of developing psychological and emotional difficulties.

Ongoing time-limited pain (chronic acute) may last for a prolonged period of time and there is a high probability that it will end once the cause is controlled or cured, such as occurs in burns pain.

Chronic non-malignant or chronic benign pain as McCaffery and Beebe (1989) point out is not benign as it is destructive (in terms of the physical, emotional and social toll that it takes on the individual, their family and their friends). Children who experience pain associated with neuralgia and rheumatoid arthritis fall into this category. McCaffery and Beebe (1989) propose a working definition of this type of pain:

> pain that has lasted six months or longer, is ongoing on a daily basis, is due to non-life-threatening causes, has not responded to currently available treatment methods, and may continue for the remainder of the patient's life. (pp. 232, 234)

Psychogenic pain (pain as a manifestation of psychiatric illness) affects a small group and although it is a very under-researched area the effect that it has on the child should not be underestimated. King (1993) states:

> Pain no matter that its cause, is what hurts . . . and deserves attention and treatment. (p. 645)

The child's actual experience of pain is modified by the context in which the pain is evoked and does not necessarily relate to actual intensity of the pain. A child who injures themselves whilst playing may experience less pain associated with that injury than a child who receives an injection whilst in hospital. The child's perceptions of their pain are modified by many factors and thus:

> Although the causal relationship between an injury and a consequent pain sensation seems direct and obvious, the pain from even such a cause is modified by a variety of factors. (McGrath, 1990, p. 21)

Eland (1988) summarizes the detrimental effects of unrelieved pain on the child as including:

- Respiratory
    Rapid shallow breathing; can lead to alkalosis
    Inadequate expansion of the lungs; bronchiectasis, atelectasis
    Inadequate cough; retention of secretions
- Cardiovascular
    Increased heart rate
    Tissue ischaemia
- Mobility
    Will not spontaneously move in bed
    Will not ambulate
- Fluid and electrolyte losses increased
    Rapid respiration and increased perspiration
    Increased metabolic rate
- Psychological consequences
    Will have nightmares about pain and surgery
    Will be less cooperative in the future for procedures
    Increased anxiety

PAIN TOLERANCE AND PAIN THRESHOLD

Pain perception/threshold is the least experience of pain that a person is able to recognize; that is, the point at which the stimulus is first felt and then the amount of pain that is subsequently felt. Pain tolerance is the intensity or duration of pain that a person is willing to endure (McCaffery and Beebe, 1989). Tolerance is often described as being high or low. People with high pain tolerances are willing to deal with intense pain or pain over a long period of time before it becomes intolerable and/or they require pain relief. The opposite is true for those people with a low tolerance for pain.

It is probably more important for the nurse to assess the child's tolerance of pain rather than assess the expected intensity or duration of pain, as it is the tolerance that is crucial to the child's experience. There is little evidence to suggest that children have a different tolerance level from adults although a study by Haslam (1969) suggests that there is a strong positive correlation between the age of the child and their pain threshold. The previously held belief that infants are incapable of experiencing/perceiving pain has now been relegated to the position of medical myth (Volpe, 1981; Booker, 1987; Anand *et al.*, 1985; McCaffery and Beebe, 1989). However, a study performed by Walco *et al.* (1990) suggests that children who had experienced repeated episodes of pain (such as those with juvenile rheumatoid arthritis and sickle cell crisis) had significantly lower pain thresholds than the healthy children in the study.

MYTHS AND MISCONCEPTIONS

The number of myths and misconceptions that abound about children and their pain reflects the previous dearth of research throughout the subject. It is only since the 1970s that the area has attracted any level of interest. The lack of scientific background allowed, if not encouraged, poor practice to continue in respect to all aspects of assessment, care and management. Prior to this, children and particularly infants were operated on, sutured, injected and subjected to intense levels of procedural pain with little, if any, consideration being given to their pain management needs. In a medical culture where the dominant feeling was that infants felt no pain and children experienced a different, less intense quality of pain from their adult counterparts abuse of the child's right to be pain free was consistently ignored. However, there is now evidence to refute many of these old myths (Table 1.1) and gradually practice is changing as a result of recent research studies and more importantly a philosophical shift to the point where all members of the multidisciplinary team involved in pain management question traditional practices and basically 'dodgy knowledge'.

Table 1.1 Misconceptions and evidence about pain in children and infants (developed from Burr, 1987, and Whaley and Wong, 1989, p. 587)

Misconception/fallacy	Facts/evidence
Neonates/infants cannot remember	Neonates may be able to remember pain and this may lead to long-term sequelae (Fitzgerald and Anand, 1993)
Neonates/infants are incapable of experiencing pain due to immaturity of their central nervous system	Volpe (1981) demonstrated that myelination is not required for pain perception. Neonates exhibit behavioural, physiological and hormonal responses to pain (Anand *et al.*, 1985; Owens and Todt, 1984; Franck 1986)
Neonates cannot cognitively appreciate pain	Booker (1987) proposes that the neonate may be able to perceive pain at the cortical level
Children and infants experience less pain than adults	Younger children may perceive a greater intensity of pain than older children (Fowler-Kerry and Lander, 1987)
Infants' and children's behaviour accurately reflects their pain	Sleeping children (Hawley, 1984) and children who are playing/are active (Eland, 1985) may be experiencing pain but coping with it (McCaffery, 1979; Eland 1985)
Children cannot describe and/or locate their pain	Children as young as 3 years have used self-report tools (Beyer and Wells, 1989) and can locate their pain (Eland and Anderson, 1977)
Children do not want to be involved in their pain management	Eland (1981) showed that a level of autonomy increased a child's feeling of control
The use of opioids causes respiratory depression and addiction	No greater risk for children and adolescents in terms of addiction (Porter and Jick, 1989)
	Dilworth and MacKellar (1987) showed no incidences of addiction in postoperative children
	'Fear of creating opioid addiction should never be a reason for withholding opioid analgesics from anyone who needs them for pain relief' (McCaffery and Wong, 1993, p. 305)
	The risk of respiratory depression is no greater in children than in adults provided the dose is appropriate

Table 1.1 contd.

Children will be truthful about their pain	Children will often withdraw when coping with pain and may not admit to their pain. Fear of what will happen next may prevent them from disclosing the truth (Mather and Mackie, 1983)
Injections do not hurt	Eland (1981) reported that children described the injection as the 'worst hurt'. Mather and Mackie (1983) state that children fear injections more than anything else in hospital

Each of these myths has now got strong evidence to refute it and the myth that the nurse/health professional is the expert in accurately assessing the child's pain is also refuted (Alder, 1990). The child will always be the expert about their own pain experience even if there are problems in communicating the richness, intensity and quality of that experience.

FACTORS AFFECTING THE CHILD'S EXPERIENCE OF PAIN

The child's experience of pain is influenced and modified by a great many factors that the nurse should be aware of if the attempt to manage pain is to be successful. These factors include experiential, behaviourial, emotional, physical and contextual/situational components. Temperament may also play a part in the child's response to pain (Wallace, 1989). All these factors play a part in the child's eventual understanding of, their ability to cope with and their experience of pain. The final pain experience

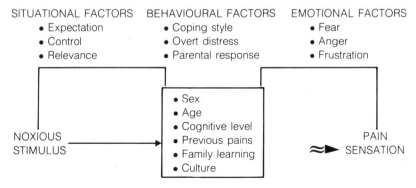

Figure 1.3 A model of the situational, behavioural and emotional factors that affect a child's pain (McGrath, 1989).

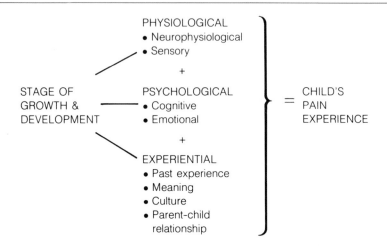

Figure 1.4 The child's pain experience (Stevens *et al.*, 1987).

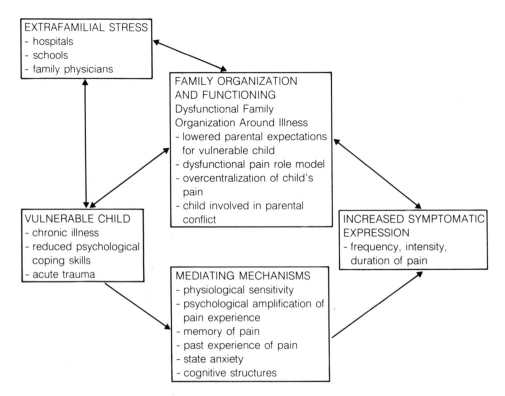

Figure 1.5 Open systems model of dysfunctional adaptation to paediatric pain (Covelman *et al.*, 1990).

is a complex response to what may have been an initial and perhaps seemingly trivial or slight noxious stimulus. McGrath (1989) and Stevens *et al.* (1987) propose models that demonstrate how a variety of internal and external factors affect the child's pain experience (see Figs 1.3 and 1.4). However, Covelman *et al.* (1990) suggest that an open systems model provides a radical departure from some traditional models related to pain since this model really attempts to understand the child in their own context and provides a guide to therapeutic intervention. The strength of this model is seen to be in the way in which a variety of therapeutic 'efforts' can be utilized to affect the child, family and their responses to the child's pain (Fig. 1.5). However, this model still requires further testing in practice.

NEONATAL MEMORY OF PAIN

Although it is recognized that children can and do remember their pain experiences and learn from modifying their responses to subsequent episodes, there is a greater level of controversy about whether or not neonates can remember pain either in the short or in the longer term. Until relatively recently the consensus was that neonates were unable to remember pain; this was due to a variety of reasons, including an immature nervous system. However, there is now an increasing amount of evidence to suggest that infants can remember pain. Chamberlain (1989) reports the memory of pain experienced by his granddaughter in the delivery room. His 29-year-old granddaughter was hypnotized and remembered that she was placed on some metal scales that were 'so straight and so hard against my back. And I'm screaming because its so painful! I am screaming and screaming and no one is coming.' Chamberlain (1989) acknowledges such reports are new but gives several other examples that support a long-term memory of very early pain experiences, including both birth experiences and circumcision pain.

Porter (1989) writes that young infants can demonstrate memories of sensory events over relatively long periods of time. She further reports an unpublished piece of work (Porter and Marshall) suggesting that mothers of infants who have required neonatal intensive care say that:

> their infants seem to have a higher threshold for subsequent pain and a lower tendency to report pain than siblings not exposed to early pain.
> (Porter, 1989, p. 551)

Tyler (1988) also supports the view that neonates do remember pain by learning through the mechanism of habituation, classical conditioning and operant conditioning. However, this is yet another area that requires further research. Despite the fact that other sensory learning does take place there is no clear evidence as yet that a memory for pain exists under 6 months of age (Johnson, 1993).

COGNITIVE DEVELOPMENT AND THE UNDERSTANDING OF PAIN

Warni (1990) describes pain as a complex 'cognitive–developmental phenomenon' and this aspect of pain needs careful consideration by the nurse. Children's understanding of their pain parallels their understanding of illness in general. As children grow and develop their ability to understand more about themselves also evolves and this developing understanding has huge implications in respect to pain management. Eiser and Patterson's (1983) study reflects children's developing understanding of their bodies and the functions that various organs perform. The children, aged 6, 8, 10 and 12 years old, were asked to draw circles on outline bodies to locate brain, heart, stomach, kidneys, liver, lungs and bladder, and to explain their function and which parts of their body they needed to eat, breathe, get rid of waste and swim. Explanation of function increased with age although interconnection concepts were not really even grasped by the 12-year-olds. This would suggest that many children have little grasp of the anatomy and physiology of their body, which means that explanations to children must be made ensuring that this is realized by the nurse.

As children develop their ability to handle concepts also increases and again this is an important factor that the nurse must take into consideration when explaining to the child about their pain, illness and procedures that are a necessary part of their treatment and care. Children's cognitive development does not always match their chronological age and it is important to consider and assess the cognitive level when talking to the child. In a study of 5–13-year-old chronically sick, hospitalized children's understanding of the cause of their illness, Brewster (1982) found that children's responses could be classified into a three-stage sequence of conceptual development. The under-7-year old children felt that illness was caused by a human action, the 7–10-year-olds thought that there was a physical cause of their illness, whereas the older children had a more complex concept of their illness and thought that it resulted from many causes and by an interaction of events.

Interestingly, children in a study undertaken by Savedra et al.(1982) showed that children who were hospitalized described their pain differently from non-hospitalized children and causes of pain were seen to be more related to hospital-linked pains.

The three-stage sequence of development described by Brewster (1982) has parallels with children's understanding of pain, as can be seen by Gaffney and Dunn's (1986) study which provided three stages in defining pain as a concept. The study focused on 680 children (5–14 years old) who were given a sentence completion task relating to aspects of pain.

- Concrete definitions: pain was defined by location or unpleasant physical properties or in terms of association with an illness (5–7 years).
- Semi-abstract definitions: pain was defined in relation to feelings or sensations. Pain was described in terms of its qualities such as 'ache' and 'sore' (8–10 years).
- Abstract definitions: pain was defined in physiological and psychological terms or as a mix of both. It was seen as having a strong emotional content and to have a purpose (11 years).

The study demonstrated that children's concepts of pain follows a developmental sequence that reflects Piaget's theory.

McGrath (1990) reports studies by Katz *et al.* (1980) and Jay *et al.* (1983) demonstrating that children's responses to pain are linked to cognitive development. Young children were seen to demonstrate more behavioural distress than older children during invasive medical procedures. Behaviour such as crying and withdrawing decreased dramatically when the children were about 7 years old, which is the age at which concrete operational thinking develops in Piagetian theory.

PIAGETIAN THEORY

Piaget's theory of cognitive development proposes four major stages in the development of logical thinking. It demonstrates how children learn to understand the world by learning to reason abstractly, think logically and to organize intellectual functions or performances. The goal of cognitive development is to attain equilibration (state of relative equilibrium). This is achieved through organization (biological way in which the infant is organized) and adaptation (means by which organization is achieved). Adaptation occurs through the processes of assimilation (taking in information; and making a map or schema in the brain which can subsequently be amended) and accommodation (means by which new information is adjusted to fit an existing schema). The four major stages of Piaget's theory are sensorimotor, preoperational, concrete operational and formal operational.

- *Sensorimotor stage (birth to 2 years).* Simple reflex responses to purposeful manipulation of the environment. Basic understanding of cause and effect, problem solving and imitation.
- *Preoperational stage (2–7 years).* The child finds difficulty in distinguishing real from unreal, and magical thinking abounds. Children tend to interpret events and objects in terms of their relationship with them to their use to them. In this stage children lack the ability to generalize about things

or to make deductions. This means that the child may not realize the need to complain formally about their pain in order to get relief from it. This has been noted by Eland and Anderson (1977). Children in this stage are also more likely to be concerned with surface features of illness and pain, which may explain their predisposition for plasters and bandages to cover up the cause (Beales, 1983). Since this stage finds difficulty in distinguishing cause from effect the child may see no connection between an analgesic injection and the subsequent relief of pain.

- *Concrete operations (7–11 years)*. Thought becomes increasingly logical; the child is able to sort, classify and organize objects and concepts. They are able to handle more than one aspect of a situation. Reasoning becomes inductive. Children in this stage will be able to relate their sensation of pain to the fact that it makes them unhappy or cross.
- *Formal operations (12–15 years)*. Abstract thought is possible and true logical thinking is present. Hypotheses can be developed and the child can philosophize over issues. Children in this stage can understand more of the physiological processes occurring and will think more deeply about what their pain means.

Castiglia (1992) suggests that Piaget's theory is not always accepted; other theories such as Erikson's theory is based on eight stages suggesting that resolution of the crisis of each stage is required to prepare for the success in subsequent stages (Erikson, 1968).

CULTURE, ETHNICITY AND PAIN

The issue of how culture modifies a child's reactions to pain is one of increasing interest although there is relatively little research available to provide hard information. Of equal interest must be the impact that culture has on the nurse's perceptions of that child's pain. Martinelli (1987) suggests that 'health care providers are often ethnocentric'. Bernstein and Pachter (1993) propose four theories/areas which suggest that pain experience is influenced by culture: individuals vary in perception and response to seemingly similar noxious stimuli; cognitive (psychological) factors and underlying attitudes change the individual's experience of pain; individuals have different 'explanatory models' of illness and 'cultural considerations' of illness; and learning from family and society influences behavioural responses to pain.

Studies that exist related to children, culture and pain pose similar problems to those in adults as it is problematic in distinguishing culture from race and deciding which is a determinant of response. In some instances pain and culture may be very closely associated, especially when responses and behaviours are closely identified with the rules and traditions of a society. Ngugi (1986) writes of belief systems within African tribes which are culturally determined. The Kikuyu or Masai man is expected to be quiet and dignified in response to pain whilst the woman can cry or act in any manner she wants to, except during labour when stoicism is required. The Luo tribe, however, allows males to wail with pain.

The studies on culture and pain response have mostly been carried out in America; Zborowski's (1952, 1969) study on 'Old Americans' (white, Anglo-Saxon Protestants with a history of three generations living in the USA), Italians, Jews and Irish is an early example. The results of the study showed differences in behaviours in seeking help for their pain, and in their pain behaviours and attitudes. Hospital staff most approved of the 'Old Americans' who were generally optimistic, unemotional in their descriptions of their pain, and would withdraw when the pain was severe. The Italian patients were more depressed with pain and frank in their expression of pain, the Irish were concerned with the future but stoical in their handling of pain and the Jewish patients sought help, sympathy and second opinions. The inference from this is that approval by the hospital staff reflected their expectations from the dominant culture as to what were appropriate responses to pain.

Lipton and Marbach's (1984) study looked at responses by blacks, Irish, Jews, Puerto Ricans and Italians in response to facial pain and found that the ethnic groups had both 'inter-ethnic homogeneity' (similar responses) and 'intra-ethnic heterogeneity' (factors that influenced the way that they responded were different).

Abu-Saad (1984) used semi-structured interviews that looked at causes, colours, descriptions, feelings about pain, coping mechanisms and positive aspects of pain in 24 children aged 9–12 years. The children came from three cultural groups: Latin-American, Asian-American and Arab-American. Very few differences were found although Arab-American and Latin-American children tended to use more sensory words when describing their pain whilst the Asian-American children used affective and evaluative words. Children in this study displayed a range of coping strategies, with medicine being the prime choice by both boys and girls in all groups. Abu-Saad (1984) concludes:

It may be crucial to be sensitive to cultural clues about pain, but it is essential not to overemphasize them. (p. 195)

Abu-Saad (1990) reports the development of a multidimensional pain assessment tool including words that Dutch children use to describe pain and suggests strongly that pain instruments should be culturally specific. Banoub-Baddour and Laryea (1991) propose that nurses should see the child as an individual within a cultural group and that a multicultural approach is important. Despite the general lack of information available it is expected that children will reflect both their families' expectations and society's expectation in their responses to pain and it may be difficult, as stated earlier, to unravel ethnicity and culture. Bernstein and Pachter (1993) suggest that a 'culturally sensitive' approach is used when caring for or researching the child in pain.

COPING STRATEGIES

Initially in this section the spontaneous coping strategies that children use in response to a painful episode will be examined rather than the strategies that they can be taught to help them cope with and manage their pain. These spontaneous strategies are important as they give added meaning to the behaviours that some children may display. Elliot and Olsen (1982) suggest that children do not engage in effective coping strategies during painful procedures unless they are prompted or guided by an adult. Jay *et al.* (1983) report that some children display extreme anticipatory behavioural distress and anxiety prior to invasive medical procedures. This behaviour, although stressful for the health professional, may seem to be a more expected reaction than some of the other coping behaviours, such as sleeping or playing, that children use to give them some degree of control over their experience (Eland and Anderson, 1977; Gross and Gardner, 1980; McCaffery, 1982).

Infant pain-coping strategies are also difficult to distinguish from general stress-coping strategies although Brazelton (1979) sees pain as another additional form of sensory input. He suggests that neonates need an appropriate amount of stimuli but that too much, especially in the preterm infant, can cause overloading and that pain may be a major factor in inducing neonatal stress. He suggests that infants cope with this by 'shutting off' from certain stimuli in an effort (cognitive or otherwise) to reduce their stress level. He warns that in these situations talking to or touching the infant can simply add to the stress load.

Emde *et al.* (1971) report a conservation withdrawal pattern that is characterized by prolonged sleeping and inactivity with no rapid eye movement (REM) sleep. Conservation withdrawal appears to occur as a result of the sensory threshold being altered to decrease the amount of sensory stimulation perceived. Painful episodes resulted in prolonged, inactive sleep.

Broome *et al.* (1990) report an unpublished study based on Rose's coping assessment tool (Savedra and Tesler, 1981) that examined coping behaviours in children in respect to preoperative injections and their behaviours after discharge. The children mostly displayed passive coping behaviours prior to injection, passive and active during the injection and mostly passive after the injection. Rose's coping assessment tool categorizes behaviours as inactive precoping or orienting, co-operative, resistive and attempting to control.

In Broome *et al.*'s (1990) study of children with cancer and their coping behaviours in respect to lumbar puncture it was found that many children saw the pre-procedure phase as a minor threat. However, during the cleansing phase the group was equally divided between active and passive behaviours. Most of the children were restrained by the nurse and unable to see the needle and many tried to find out what was happening. The numbing phase evoked an increase in active behaviours such as kicking and screaming. The children displayed more inactive behaviours during the actual lumbar puncture stage and were generally quiet and withdrawn. The children who were mostly passive appeared to recover quickly and started to interact more frequently. Behavioural studies such as this are important in ascertaining how children cope and what type of interventions would be appropiate, such as providing good preparatory information prior to and during the procedure so that the child understands what is happening and what is about to happen.

Blount *et al.* (1991) studied 22 children (5–13 years) with cancer and found that those children categorized as high copers had parents who adopted 'coping-promoting' behaviours and that the high coping children responded well to coping prompts. Ross and Ross (1984) in a study of school-aged children found that only a minority of children initiated the use of their coping strategies, such as clenching their fists and using distraction.

Other spontaneous coping strategies that have been examined are shown in a study by Brown *et al.* (1986) which showed that children responded to dental pain by displaying either coping or catastrophizing strategies. Spontaneous coping responses included telling themselves that they could cope with it, thinking of something else or listening to music, relaxation or thought stopping. The catastrophizing responses/strategies included focusing on the negative aspects of the situation, thinking of escaping and avoiding the situation, worries about unlikely unpleasant consequence and concerns about the dentist. The majority of children in this study were categorized as catastrophizers.

ETHICAL ISSUES

Ethical issues related to pain and the child should be a prime consideration of all members of the multidisciplinary team and those involved in research. Many ethically based questions arise in relation to children's pain, including: undertreatment of pain; using placebos; not involving the child in the management of their pain; disbelieving the child's reports of pain; involving children in painful procedures without gaining their consent; and involving children in research studies. There are no easy answers to these issues but the child has the right to be central to all considerations and decisions and the role of the nurse is central to this as well. This right is internationally recognized. UNICEF in their Declaration of the Rights of the Child state:

Principle 8
The child shall in all circumstances be among the first to receive protection and relief.
Principle 9
The child shall be protected from all forms of neglect, cruelty and exploitation.

The Charter for Children in Hospital (Action for Sick Children, formerly NAWCH) states that:

Children and/or their parents shall have the right to information appropriate to age and understanding.

Children and/or their parents shall have the right to informed participation in all decisions involving their health care. Every child shall be protected form unnecessary medical treatment and steps taken to mitigate physical or emotional distress.

One issue that needs consideration in respect to children's involvement in research studies is whether or not 'voluntariness', which is a central issue to all research, can be achieved if the subject is a child. Brykczńska (1989) states:

A child must prove that he or she is aware of the concept of voluntariness and of his or her own free will wishes to participate and all this on the basis of informed consent . . . a tall order for adults, let alone a child. (p. 120)

It is questionable how voluntary a child is in respect to their admission to a study. Their consent should never be taken for granted and the child's individual 'best interests' must always be at the forefront. One study that perhaps did not understand the child's best interests was that performed by Smith (1985), who decided that only minimal harm resulted to healthy children involved in having blood samples taken. Since only minimal harm resulted it was considered an ethically acceptable undertaking. However, considering the work by researchers on the attitudes and responses that children have to venipuncture and injection pain this must be questioned. Work by Mather and Mackie (1989) suggests that children tend to prefer moderately severe postoperative pain to an analgesic injection, and Eland and Anderson (1977) reported that many children find that 'needles or shots' are the most painful part of a hospital admission.

Brykczńska (1989) cites Redmon (1986), who feels that children can be used as subjects in non-therapeutic research since that participation is part of their 'learning and growing experience'. A further voice is added to this contentious issue as McGrath (1993) states that:

pain research should be regarded as a special and valued collaboration between the investigators and children (and their parents or guardians) . . . The probable benefits (direct and indirect) for a child's participation must exceed any potential harm. (p. 56)

McGrath (1993) further eloquently argues that provided the study has scientific value, that the research methodology is sound, the research is justified and that benefit to children in general outweighs the discomfort experienced by the individual children in a study then induced pain may be acceptable and a needed part of the ongoing research programme into children's pain. Perhaps the difficulty with this argument, despite its obvious merits, is in the ability to design a methodology and study that is totally beyond reproach.

Lack of treatment or undertreatment of a child's pain is an area of major concern since many health care professionals tend to veer towards protecting themselves from the consequences of administering analgesia rather than protecting the child from the almost inevitable deleterious consequences of pain. There is an increasing body of evidence demonstrating that proactive treatment is the only ethical route to take in pain prevention and management. The morbidity and possible mortality associated with non-management is something which is not ethically acceptable. Additionally the emotional trauma experienced by both the child and their family is another area that requires ethical consideration. Lawson (1986) in a letter to the editor of *Birth* writes of her very premature son who had undergone a 90-minute period of major surgery without any form of pain relief or anaesthesia. The explanation offered was that 'it has never been demonstrated that babies can feel pain'. Lawson stated that 'what happened to my son meets the dictionary definition of vivisection'.

Placing pain control at or near the bottom of nursing priorities (Burokas, 1985) again is ethically unacceptable. Stevens *et al.* (1987) highlight this issue when they state:

> Often more concrete responsibilities such as fluid and electrolyte balance and fever control often preempt pain management as a nursing priority even though pain may be the most pressing concern of the child and/or the family. (pp. 162–163)

Children have the right to give consent and therefore the right to withhold consent.

> The rights of the children to give consent to treatment were reinforced by a judgement in the House of Lords in 1985 [the Gillick case] which stated that the parental right to determine whether or not their minor child below the age of 16 years will have medical treatments terminates if and when the child achieves sufficient understanding and intelligence to enable him or her to fully understand what is proposed. (Department of Health, 1991)

Douglas (1993) states that

> Once consent has been given the issue becomes one of how to help the child cope with the stress of the event, rather than one of imposing procedures on a struggling child. (p. 176)

Children have the right to a feeling of security and to be nursed in an atmosphere of trust and caring; providing good pain management is one way in which this can be fulfilled. Trust relies on the child being secure and this implies that they will not be deceived by the use of placebos when the health professional suspects that the child's pain is not 'real'. The use of placebos is unethical and does not even begin to address the issue of what is causing the child to complain of pain. The child must be believed even in the absence of an organic explanation for the pain.

THE CHILD'S FAMILY

The child's family is paramount in ensuring that their pain experience is managed effectively. The child's parents can act as a buffer between the child and the hospital environment (Wallace, 1989). The parents and siblings can be stressed by the child's pain and they may experience feelings of helplessness, guilt, anger and depression (Alexander et al., 1986). Again this is an area that is worthy of further research. Parents may feel inadequate or unsure of how best to care for their child during painful procedures (Miles and Carter, 1982). Family-centred care is important if pain is to be managed appropriately. Children need their family and when they are in pain they perhaps need them even more. Children's nurses must respect this fundamental need and be willing to acknowledge the resource that the family represents and work with them. Dearmun (1993) proposes that the potential of the parents to contribute to the total care of their child should not be underestimated. However, she rightly warns that:

> Their involvement should be fully negotiated, not foisted upon them through expediency or lack of nursing resources. (p. 9)

Shelton et al. (1987) propose a framework of family-centred care that enshrines many of the principles upon which good pain management is built (Table 1.2).

Table 1.2 A framework of family-centred care

1.	Recognition that the family is the constant in the child's life while the service systems and personnel within those systems fluctuate
2.	Facilitation of parent/professional collaboration at all levels of health care
3.	Sharing of unbiased and complete information with parents about their child's care on an ongoing basis in an appropriate and supportive manner
4.	Implementation of appropriate policies and programmes that are comprehensive and provide emotional and financial support to meet families' needs
5.	Recognition of family strengths, and individuality and respect of different methods of coping
6.	Understanding and incorporating the developmental and emotional needs of infants, children and adolescents and their families into health care delivery systems.
7.	Encouragement and facilitation of parent-to-child support
8.	Assurance that the design of health care delivery systems is flexible, accessible and responsive to family needs

The family also provides the environment in which most children learn how to cope with and respond to pain. Parental expectations will often depend on and reflect the child's age, gender and birth order. The family provides a powerful means of enculturation in respect to pain (Mathews *et al.*, 1993). Families may find it difficult themselves to 'live up' to their own expectation about pain.

The family should be acknowledged as a rich resource in terms of helping to deal with the child's experiences – despite the fact that some studies demonstrate that nurses do not rely on the parents' input (O'Brien and Konsler, 1988) or feel threatened by the presence of parents during difficult pain-invoking procedures (Goodall, 1979). It is important to remember that in Ross and Ross's (1984) study 99.2% of the children (5–12 years old) surveyed said that the presence of their parents would have been the most helpful thing when they were experiencing their worst pain. Further studies have demonstrated the crucial role of parents in supporting their children (Dearmun, 1991; Webb *et al.*, 1986). Some studies suggest that a reduction in parental stress can result in similar reductions in the child's level of stress (Vardaro, 1978; Jay *et al.*, 1983). This is partly supported by the study undertaken by Whitsett and Hagen (1990).

Some parents are anxious about the use of powerful analgesics and these fears need to be allayed to allow the child to have the opportunity to be pain free (Schechter, 1989). Others may not think it necessary to tell the nurse that they feel their child is in need of analgesia since they think that the nurse is aware of what is needed and will administer it (Eland, 1988). Mills (1989) reports that parents feel that nurses are 'more experienced' in respect to pain assessment and therefore they may not report pain to them.

McCaffery and Beebe (1989) emphasize the key role of the child's family (including grandparents) in helping the child. They state:

> For the benefit of both the child of any age and his parents, allow the parents to be with, touch, and hold the child to the extent possible without causing undue distress for either. (p. 269)

This can be managed through skilled nursing care in supporting the family, teaching them strategies for caring for the child and helping them to manage their own distress.

The family should be involved primarily by discussing their child's pain with them as this gives the nurses insight into the child's own individual needs, fears, coping behaviours and experiences and helps the parents to identify ways in which they can help. McCaffery and Beebe (1989) provide a Parent Interview Schedule which aims to provide information about the child's pain, to increase the parents' ability to assess and relieve their child's pain and finally involvement in providing comfort and relief (Fig. 1.6). This involvement is crucial in ensuring that parents do not feel they have no role to play and have no control over their child's care. It is recommended that the

Parent Interview Regarding Child's Pain/Hurt

Child: _____ Parent/Caregiver: _____ Date:_____

1. Total Current Situation

What are your major concerns (unrelated to pain), if any, about the current situation/hospitalization in general, e.g., finances, care of other children, cause or seriousness of illnesses?

What are your child's major concerns (unrelated to pain), if any, about the current situation/hospitalization in general, e.g. being separated from parent, sleeping in a different bed or room, missing a birthday party, school work?

II. Child's Previous Experiences with Pain/Hurt

What types of pain has your child had before? Include descriptions of cause, duration, severity, frequency, and other important aspects.

What words, if any, does your child use for pain or hurt?

How does your child usually act when he is *suddenly* hurt, e.g., falls down?

How does your child usually act when he has been *hurting for a long time*, e.g., with a sore throat or earache?

III. Assessment of the Child's Current Pain

Since no one but the child knows if he hurts, the health team needs your help in finding out when your child is hurting and whether or not efforts to relieve the pain are working.

What behaviors indicate that your child is or is not in pain right now? For example, can you get your child to smile at you?

A written record, called a "Flow Sheet" can be very helpful. What do you suggest be recorded on the flow sheet?

List of behaviors that probably indicate pain:

List of behaviors that probably indicate comfort:

Parent Interview Regarding Child's Pain/Hurt – cont'd.

IV. Comforting the Child and/or Relieving the Pain

When your child hurts, what do you usually do to comfort your child or relieve the pain? Which work best? Which could you do now?

When your child hurts, what does the child do for himself that seems to help? How can we help the child help himself?

Considering the pain your child has now or will have, what are your concerns about being with your child while he is hurting or is having a painful procedure?

What would you like to learn about how you can soothe or distract your child during pain?

If painful procedures are performed, do you wish to be with your child? If this varies, during which procedures do you wish to be present and which ones would you rather avoid?

Do you have any ideas about how far in advance your child would like to be informed about a painful procedure?

Other Comments

Is there anything special we should know about your child and pain? Is there anything disturbing to the child that we should *not* do?

• May be duplicated for use in clinical practice. From McCaffery, M. and Beeve, A: PAIN: CLINICAL MANUAL FOR NURSING PRACTICE, St. Louis, 1989, The CV Mosby Company.

Figure 1.6 (with permission)

nurse interviews both parents to elicit a comprehensive amount of information. In an interview (by the author) with the parents of a 14-month-old girl they emphasized the need to be informed and the trust that they placed in the nursing and medical staff:

> I tend to trust the nurses' judgement about the pain relief – they have always done alright by Chloe – we are here for emotional support as much as anything . . . we cope because we're very strong together . . . When the anaesthetist spoke to us last night I think that's actually the first time it [pain] has ever been addressed since she's been in here . . . she's been in under the needle a few times now and pain management was never discussed but here [ward] they talked about what would happen during the operation and that she'd be OK when she came back because they'd give her so and so and it was nice to know . . . yes it made a real difference – we felt better about her going for the operation. (Chloe's parents. Chloe, aged 14 months, had undergone multiple admissions requiring intensive care, and many invasive procedures)

Another approach involves parents by using the Pain Experience Inventory (Hester and Barcus, 1986), which also provides a series of questions for parents (and the child).

Watt-Watson et al.'s (1990) study on parents' perceptions of their child's experiences of acute pain found that they readily identified pain behaviours and they suggest that pain measurement tools could be used by the parents. They also identified that parents felt the need for more information about the painful procedures, including the length of time the child would experience the pain. Most parents in this study wanted to stay with their child although some felt that they did not know what they could do to help. Interestingly, and worryingly, one mother responded by saying:

> I'm afraid to tell the doctors about his pain because I know it will mean more tests. (Watt-Watson et al., 1990, p. 346)

Understanding that parents may feel trapped by their child's pain is important. Another worrying issue that was highlighted by this study was the rejection and distress that those parents who were asked to leave their child during the procedure experienced. The study concludes that parental involvement should be encouraged so they can take a more active role in comforting their child.

This feeling of needing to be involved is echoed by other parents, and parents should be seen as a vital resource and their involvement should be encouraged and supported. Shelley (1993) speaking on behalf of Action for Sick Children (ASC) states:

> If doctors and nurses are confused about pain in children they are in danger of undermining parents' instincts about their own child. (p. 5)

Parents need to be involved throughout their child's encounter with the health care system and this means that information will be needed from the initial contact, probably in the community, throughout any hospital admission and then when they return home. Information will be needed in both the verbal and written form.

NURSES' ROLE: OVERVIEW

Children's nurses have a key role in ensuring that children who require nursing care experience a caring and safe environment in which they feel secure and comfortable. The experience of pain can readily undermine that atmosphere of care and trust as the nurse is often a key person involved either in the procedure that creates the pain or in their care whilst they experience pain. The nurse is pivotal in the management of pain and has a multiplicity of roles, all of which should be child oriented (Fig. 1.7).

Pain prevention and management must be seen as a priority of care, and in developing any plan of nursing care the nurse is obliged to ensure that pain receives a high degree of attention. The nurse must assess, document, evaluate and act upon the child's pain and ensure that if the treatment is ineffective in controlling the child's pain an alternative approach (or approaches) is taken.

The nurse must act as an advocate for the child (Thyer, 1992) and remember that they are personally accountable for their practice and that they should always act to promote and safeguard the child and ensure that no act or

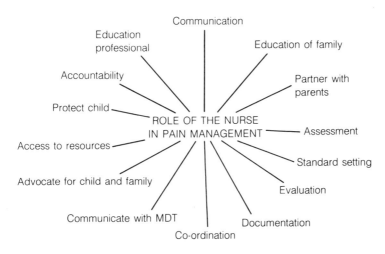

Figure 1.7 Role of the nurse.

omission is detrimental to the client's interests (UK Central Council for Nursing, Midwifery and Health Visiting, 1992). The philosophy that underpins every nurse's practice must include a commitment to pain management and a commitment to work with the child and their family. Regardless of whichever model is used to provide the framework of care, pain should appear as an issue. If it does not then this should be resolved. Pain must be documented and the documentation reviewed regularly. The importance of clear documentation should not be underestimated as it is an 'integral part of care and not a distraction from its provision' (UK Central Council for Nursing, Midwifery and Health Visiting, 1993, p. 15). Assessment is ongoing as the child's pain is ongoing and dynamic. Nurses have a responsibility to learn and develop their knowledge of the many issues that impact on the child's pain.

Child-centred nursing or a family-centred approach is vital if pain management is to be successful. Dearmun (1993) suggests that the role of the nurse within the child–parent–nurse partnership is an essential component to children's nursing in general and has much to offer pain management specifically.

A vital aspect of good pain management lies in the nurse's ability to communicate with the rest of the multidisciplinary team, particularly those responsible for prescribing analgesia (Eland, 1988). Foster and Hester (1990) and Dilworth (1988) suggest that there may be many differing philosophies of pain management held by those responsible for caring for a child and that these can have a detrimental effect on the overall quality of care delivered. However, a focused, child-centred philosophy should be adopted by the team so that effective pain relief can occur. The nurse must act as the child's advocate and ensure that the analgesia prescribed is appropriate and effective. To be able to assess the effectiveness of the analgesia the nurse must consider what, when and how the analgesia has been given, what if any effect it has had, how frequently it has been used, what side-effects are being experienced (if any) and any other information felt to be appropriate.

Nurses must take a holistic approach to pain management and see it as more than simply the inevitable outcome of surgery, injections and injury. The child's previous pain experiences, cognitive level, beliefs, fears, coping strategies and preferences must be considered.

Nurses must also be pain preventers in terms of ensuring that the child is not subjected to unnecessary pain, such as repeated sessions of blood taking when 'grouping bloods' means that the child only needs one venepuncture.

Good preparation in the form of preoperative and pre-procedure teaching and discussions can help to allay the child's fears and help them to manage their pain and feel more in control. Management strategies such as imagery and distraction can be introduced at an early stage to familiarize the child with the techniques and to give them a degree of confidence in their use. If we as nurses feel the challenge of effectively and holistically managing a child's pain to be difficult it would be well for us to remember it is a whole lot tougher for the child and their family. It is the nurse's responsibility to make stringent efforts to provide holistic pain management. Nurses provide the 'cornerstone' of care for the patient in pain (McCaffery and Beebe, 1989). Deynes *et al.* (1991) highlighted a number of existing roles, including modifying the child's environment, involving the child in their care, directly caring for the child, and facilitating care and techniques. In pharmacological management four rights are held to be crucial: right drug, right dose, right route and right time. In nursing care an additional six rights need to be considered: right assessment, right technique, right preparation, right support, right information and right care (Fig. 1.8).

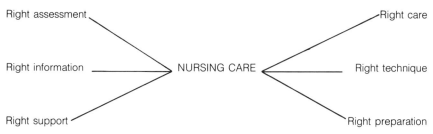

Figure 1.8 The six rights of nursing care.

REFERENCES

Abu-Saad, H. (1984) Cultural group indicators of pain in children. *Maternal Child Nursing Journal*, **13**: 187–196.

Abu-Saad, H.H. (1990) Toward the development of an instrument to assess pain in children: Dutch study. In: Tyler, D.C. and Krane, E.J. (eds), *Advances in Pain Research Therapy*, Vol. 15. Raven Press, New York, pp. 101–106.

Alder, S. (1990) Taking children at their word. *Professional Nurse*, **5**(8): 397–402.

Alexander, D., White, M. and Powell, G. (1986) Anxiety of non-rooming-in parents of hospitalized children. *Children's Health Care*, **15**(1): 14–20.

Anand, K.J.S., Brown, M.J. and Causon, R.C. (1985) Can the human neonate mount an endocrine/metabolic response to surgery? *Journal of Pediatric Surgery*, **20**: 41–48.

Banoub-Baddour, S. and Laryea, M. (1991) Children in pain: a culturally sensitive perspective for child care professionals. *Journal of Child and Youth Care*, **6**(1); 19–24.

Beales, J.G. (1983) Factors influencing the expectation of pain among patients in a children's burns unit. *Burns*, **9**: 187–192.

Bernstein, B.A. and Pachter, L.M. (1993) Cultural considerations in children's pain. In: Schechter, N.L., Berde, C.B. and Yaster, M. (eds), *Pain in Infants, Children, and Adolescents*. Williams & Wilkins, Baltimore, pp. 113–122.

Beyer, J.E. and Wells, N. (1989) The assessment of pain in children. *Pediatric Clinics of North America*, **36**: 837–854.

Blount, R.L., Landolf-Fritshe, B., Powers, S.W. and Sturges, J.W. (1991) Differences between high and low coping children and between parent and staff behaviors during painful medical procedures. *Journal of Pediatric Psychology*, **16**(6): 795–809.

Booker, P.D. (1987) Postoperative analgesia for neonates. *Anaesthesia*, **42**: 343–345.

Brazelton, T.B. (1979) Behavioural competence of the newborn. *Seminars in Perinatology*, **3**: 35–44.

Brewster, A.B. (1982) Chronically ill hospitalized children's concepts of their illness. *Pediatrics*, **69**: 355–362.

Broome, M.E., Bates, T.A., Lillis, P.P.Y. and Wilson McGahee, T. (1990) Children's medical fears, coping behaviors, and pain perceptions during a lumbar puncture. *Oncology Nursing Forum*, **17**(3): 361–367.

Brown, J.M. O'Keefe, J., Sanders, S.H. and Baker, B. (1986) Developmental changes in children's cognition to stressful and painful situations.

Brykczńska, G.M. (1989) *Ethics in Paediatric Nursing*. Chapman & Hall, London.

Burokas, L. (1985) Factors affecting nurses' decisions to medicate pediatric patients after surgery. *Heart and Lung*, **14**(4): 373–379.

Burr, S. (1987) Pain in childhood. *Nursing*, **24**: 890–896.

Castiglia, P.T. (1992) Developing a theoretical framework for growth and development. In: Castiglia, P.T. and Harbin, R.E. (eds), *Child Health Care: Process and Practice*. Lippincott, Philadelphia, pp. 57–74.

Chamberlain, D.B. (1989) Babies remember pain. *Pre- and Peri-natal Psychology*, **3**(4): 297–310.

Covelman, K., Scott, S., Buchanan, B. and Rosman, B. (1990) Pediatric pain control: a family systems model. In: Tyler, D.C. and Krane, E.J. (eds), *Advances in Pain Research Therapy*, Vol. 15. Raven Press, New York.

Dearmun, A. (1991) Perceptions of parental partnership. *Paediatric Nursing*, **4**(7): 6–10.

Dearmun, A. (1993) Towards a partnership in pain management. *Paediatric Nursing*, **5**(5): 8–10.

Deynes, M.J., Neuman, B.M. and Villarruel, A.M. (1991) Nursing actions to prevent and alleviate pain in hospitalized children. *Issues in Comprehensive Pediatric Nursing*, **14**(1): 31–48.

Dilworth, N.M. (1988) Children in pain: an underprivileged group. *Journal of Pediatric Surgery*, **23**: 103–104.

Dilworth, N.M. and MacKellar, A. (1987) Pain relief for the pediatric surgical patient. *Journal of Pediatric Surgery*, **22**: 264–266.

Douglas, J. (1993) *Psychology and Nursing Children*. BPS Books and Macmillan Press, Leicester.

Eiser, C. and Patterson, D. (1983) Slugs, snails and puppy dog tails – children's ideas about the inside of their bodies. *Child Health Care Development*, **9**: 233–240.

Eland, J. (1981) Minimizing pain associated with prekindergarten intramuscular injections. *Issues in Comprehensive Pediatric Nursing*, **5**: 361–372.

Eland, J. (1985) The child who is hurting. *Seminars Oncology Nursing*, **1**: 116–122.

Eland, J.M. (1988) Persistence of pain research: one nurse researcher's efforts. *Recent Advances in Nursing*, **21**: 43–62.

Eland, J.M. and Anderson, J.E. (1977) The experience of pain in children. In: Jacox, A. (ed.), *Pain: A Source Book for Nurses and Health Professionals*. Little, Brown & Co., Boston, pp. 453–473.

Elliot, C.H. and Olsen, R.A. (1982) The management of children's behavioural distress in response to painful medical treatment for burn injuries. Paper presented at a meeting of the American Psychology Association, Washington, DC. Cited in Burr, S. (1987) Pain in childhood. *Nursing*, **24**, 890–896.

Emde, R.N., Harmon, R.J., Metcalf, D. *et al.* (1971) Stress and neonatal sleep *Psychosomatic Medicine*, **33**: 491–497.

Erikson, E.H. (1968) *Childhood and Society*. Norton, New York.

Fitzgerald, M. and Anand, K.J.S. (1993) Developmental neuroanatomy and neurophysiology of pain. In: Schechter, N.L., Berde, C.B. and Yaster, M. (eds), *Pain in Infants, Children, and Adolescents*. Williams & Wilkins, Baltimore, pp. 11–31.

Foster, R.L. and Hester, N.O. (1990) The relationship between pain ratings and pharmacologic interventions for children in pain. In: Tyler, D.C. and Krane, E.J. *Advances in Pain Research Therapy*, Vol. 15. Raven Press, New York, pp. 31–36.

Fowler-Kerry, S. and Lander, J.R. (1987) Management of injection pain in children. *Pain*, **30**: 169–175.

Franck, L.S. (1986) A new method to quantitatively describe pain behavior in infants. *Nursing Research*, **35**(1): 28–31.

Gaffney, A. and Dunn, E.A. (1986) Developmental aspects of children's definitions of pain. *Pain*, **26**: 105–117.

Goodall, A. (1979) Perception's of nurses towards parent's participation on pediatric oncology units. *Cancer Nursing*, **2**(1): 38–46.

Gross, S. and Gardner, G. (1980) Child pain: treatment approaches. In: Smith, W., Merskey, H. and Gross, S. (eds), *Pain: Meaning and Management*. SP Medical & Scientific Books, New York.

Haslam, D. (1969) Age and perception of pain. *Psychonomic Science*, **15**: 86.

Hawley, D.D. (1984) Postoperative pain in children: misconceptions, descriptions and interventions. *Pediatric Nursing*, **10**: 20–23.

Hester, N. and Barcus, C. (1986) Assessment and management of pain in children. *Pediatrics: Nursing Update*, **1**(14): 3.

Jay, S.M., Ozolins, M., Elliott, C.H. and Caldwell, S. (1983) Assessment of children's distress during painful medical procedures. *Health Psychology*, **2**: 133–147.

Johnston, C. (1993) Development of psychological responses to pain in infants and toddlers. In: Schechter, N.L., Berde, C.B. and Yaster, M. (eds), *Pain in Infants, Children, and Adolescents*. Williams & Wilkins, Baltimore, pp. 65–74.

Justins, D.M. (1991) Pain relief. In Adams, A.P. and Cashman, J.N. (eds), *Anaesthesia, Analgesia, and Intensive Care*. Edward Arnold, London, pp. 263–278.

Katz, E.R., Kellerman, J. and Siegel, S.E. (1980) Behavioral distress in children with cancer undergoing medical procedures: developmental consideration. *Journal of Consulting and Clinical Psychology*, **48**: 356–365. Cited in McGrath, P.A. (1990) *Pain in Children: Nature, Assessment and Treatment*. Guilford Press, New York.

King, S.R. (1993) Somatoform pain. In: Schechter, N.L., Berde, C.B., and Yaster, M.

(eds), *Pain in Infants, Children, and Adolescents*. Williams & Wilkins, Baltimore, pp. 639–647.

Lawson, J.R. (1986) Letter to the Editor. *Birth*, **13**: 124–125.

Lipton, J.A. and Marbach, J.J. (1984) Ethnicity and the pain experience. *Social Science and Medicine*, **19**(12): 1279–1298.

Martinelli, A.M. (1987) Pain and ethnicity: how people of different cultures experience pain. *AORN Journal*, **46**(2): 273–274, 276, 278, 280–281.

Mather, L. and Mackie, J. (1983) The incidence of post-operative pain in children. *Pain*, **15**: 271–282.

Mathews, J.R., McGrath, P.J. and Pigeon, H. (1993) Assessment and measurement of pain in children: In: Schechter, N.L., Berde, C.B. and Yaster, M. (eds), *Pain in Infants, Children, and Adolescents*. Williams & Wilkins, Baltimore, pp. 97–111.

McCaffery, M. (1979) *Nursing Management of the Patient with Pain*. J.B. Lippincott, New York.

McCaffery, M. (1982) Pain control in children. In: Henning, J.S. (ed.), *The Rights of Children*. Thomas, Springfield, IL.

McCaffery, M. and Beebe, A. (1989) *Pain Clinical Manual for Nursing Practice*. Mosby, St. Louis.

McCaffery, M. and Wong, D.L. (1993) Nursing interventions for pain control in children. In: Schechter, N.L., Berde, C.B. and Yaster, M. (eds), *Pain in Infants, Children, and Adolescents*. Williams & Wilkins, Baltimore, pp. 295–316.

McGrath, P.A. (1989) Evaluating a child's pain. *Journal of Pain and Symptom Management*, **4**: 192–214.

McGrath, P.A. (1990) *Pain in Children: Nature, Assessment and Treatment*. Guilford Press, New York.

McGrath, P.A. (1993) Inducing pain in children: a controversial issue. *Pain*, **52**: 255–257.

Merskey, H. (1986) Classification of chronic pain. *Pain* (Suppl.) **3**: S1–S225.

Miles, M. and Carter, M. (1982) Sources of parental stress in pediatric intensive care units. *Children's Health Care*, **11**(3): 65–69.

Mills, N.M. (1989) Acute pain behaviour in infants and toddlers: In: Funk, S.G. *et al.* (eds), *Key Aspects of Comfort: Management of Pain, Fatigue and Nausea*. Springer, New York, pp. 52–59.

Ngugi, E.N. (1986) Pain: an African perspective. *Nursing Practice*, **1**: 169–176.

O'Brien, S. and Konsler, G. (1988) Alleviating children's postoperative pain. *Maternal Child Nursing*, **13**(3): 183–186.

Porter, F. (1989) Pain in the newborn. *Clinics in Perinatology*, **16**(2): 549–564.

Owens, M.E. and Todt, E.H. (1984) Pain in infancy: neonatal reaction to heel lance. *Pain*, **20**: 77–86.

Porter, J. and Jick, H. (1980) Addiction rare in patients treated with narcotics. *New England Journal of Medicine*, **302**: 123.

Redmon, R.B. (1986) How children can be respected as 'ends' yet still be used as subjects in non-therapeutic research. *Journal of Medical Ethics*, **12**: 77–82. Cited in Brykczńska, G.M. (1989) *Ethics in Paediatric Nursing*. Chapman & Hall, London.

Ross, D.M. and Ross, S.A. (1984) Childhood pain: the school aged child's viewpoint. *Pain*, **20**: 179–191.

Savedra, M. and Tesler, M. (1981) Coping strategies of hospitalized school-age children. *Western Journal of Nursing Research*, **3**(4): 371–384.

Savedra, M., Gibbons, P., Tesler, M., Ward, J. and Wegner, C. (1982) How do children describe pain? A tentative assessment. *Pain*, **14**: 95–104.

Schechter, N.L. (1989) The undertreatment of pain in children: an overview. *Pediatric Clinics of North America*, **36**: 781–794.

Schechter, N.L., Berde, C.B. and Yaster, M. (1993) Pain in infants, children, and adolescents: an overview. In: Schechter, N.L., Berde, C.B. and Yaster, M. (eds), *Pain in Infants, Children, and Adolescents*. Williams & Wilkins, Baltimore, pp. 3–10.

Shelley, P. (1993) Taking action. *Nursing Standard (Suppl.)*, **7**(25): 3.

Shelton, T. *et al.* (1987) *Family Centred Care for Children with Special Healthcare Need*. Association for the Care of Children's Health, Washington.

Smith, M. (1985) Taking blood from children causes no more than minimal harm. *Journal of Medical Ethics*, **11**(3): 127–132.

Sternbach, R.A. (1968) *Pain: A Psychophysiological Analysis*. Academic Press, New York.

Stevens, B., Hunsberger, M. and Browne, G. (1987) Pain in children: theoretical, research and practice dilemmas. *Journal of Pediatric Nursing*, **2**(3): 154–166.

Thyer, S. (1992) Pediatric pain: concepts for caring. *Contemporary Nurse: A Journal for the Australian Nursing Profession*, **1**(1): 27–32.

Tyler, D.C. (1988) Pain in the neonate. *Pre and Post-natal Psychology*, **3**(1): 53–59.

UK Central Council for Nursing, Midwifery and Health Visiting (1992) *Code of Professional Conduct for the Nurse, Midwife and Health Visitor*. UKCC, London.

UK Central Council for Nursing, Midwifery and Health Visiting (1993) *Standards for Records and Record Keeping*. UKCC, London.

Vardaro, J.A. (1978) Preadmission anxiety and mother–child relationships. *Journal of Association of Care of Children in Hospital*. **7**: 8–15.

Volpe, J. (1981) *Neurology of the Newborn*, Saunders, Philadelphia.

Walco, G.A., Dampier, C.D., Hartstein, G., Djordjevic, D. and Miller, L. (1990) The relationship between recurrent clinical pain and pain threshold in children. In: Tyler, D.C. and Krane, E.J. (eds), *Advances in Pain Research Therapy*, Vol. 15. Raven Press, New York, pp. 333–340.

Wallace, M.R. (1989) Temperament: a variable in children's pain management. *Pediatric Nursing*, **15**(2): 118–121.

Warni, J.W. (1990) Behavioral management of pain in children. In: Tyler, D.C. and Krane, E.J. (eds), *Advances in Pain Research Therapy*, Vol. 15. Raven Press, New York, pp. 215–234.

Watt-Watson, J.H. Evernden, C. and Lawson, C. (1990) Parents' perceptions of their child's acute pain experience. *Journal of Pediatric Nursing*, **5**(5): 344–349.

Webb, N., Hull, D. and Madeley, R. (1985) Care by parents in hospital. *British Medical Journal*, **291**: 176–177.

Whaley, L.F. and Wong, D.L. (1989) *Essentials of Pediatric Nursing*, 3rd edn. Mosby, St Louis, p. 587.

Whitsett, S.F. and Hagen, W. (1990) Parental involvement in the behavioral management of pain in pediatric oncology patients: a preliminary evaluation. In:

Tyler, D.C. and Krane, E.J. (eds), *Advances in Pain Research Therapy*, Vol. 15. Raven Press, New York, pp. 373–382.

Zborowski, M. (1952) Cultural components in response to pain. *Journal of Social Issues*, **8**: 16–30.

Zborowski, M. (1969) *People in Pain*. Jossey-Bass, San Francisco.

An overview of pain theory | 2

INTRODUCTION

A variety of pain theories have been proposed and each has attempted to explain pain based on the available scientific literature. None of them completely explains pain and all of them have been criticized. However, the gate control theory (Melzack and Wall, 1965) is the one that is currently accepted as most adequately explaining pain perception. Understanding of the complexity of the pain experience has come a long way from the simple theory proposed by Descartes in 1644 (Fig. 2.1).

Descartes proposed what is seen as a classic specificity theory, and he used the analogy of a bell-ringing mechanism found in a church. He proposed that a noxious stimulus would excite a point in the skin which would pull a delicate cord; this cord ended in a pore which was opened when pulled. In this way the cord rang a bell in the brain to create awareness of the pain. This theory is attractive due to its simplicity and was not really questioned until medicine became more scientific in the nineteenth century. Its biggest flaw is that it does not account for the fact that a single stimulus can create different responses and emotional and cognitive issues are not considered. It is described as an early form of specificity theory (Melzack and Wall, 1988).

ANATOMY OF PAIN AND GATE CONTROL THEORY

Current understanding of pain experience is considerably more complicated than Descartes' theory and, although it provides a challenge to unravel the 'mysteries' of pain, current thinking does provide a basis for clinical intervention. Modern thinking is based on gate control theory, which was first proposed by Melzack and Wall in 1965 and although the theory does not provide all the answers it is commonly seen to inform practice fundamentally in relation to the management of pain.

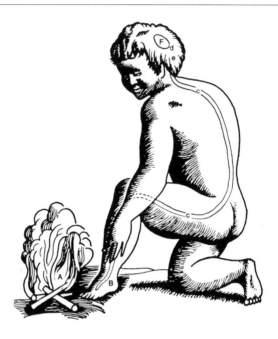

Figure 2.1 Descartes' (1664) theory of pain perception. He writes: 'If for example fire (A) comes near the foot (B), the minute particles of this fire, which as you know move with great velocity, have the power to set in motion the spot of the skin of the foot which they touch, and by this means pulling upon the delicate thread (cc) which is attached to the spot of the skin, they open up at the same instant the pore (de) against which the delicate thread ends, just as by pulling at one end of a rope one makes to strike at the same instant a bell which hangs at the other end.' Reproduced from Melzack, R. and Wall, P.D. (1988) *The Challenge of Pain*, 2nd edn, by permission of the publishers Penguin Books.

Pain transmission is stimulated by injured tissue. Barasi (1991) states that:

It is not entirely clear how the receptor converts the noxious stimuli into an electrical signal (i.e., the action potential). (p. 2)

However, there is a process whereby release of injured tissue products results in the stimulation of pain transmission. Injured tissue releases products including the very potent bradykinin, substance P (which stimulates the release of histamine from the mast cells), acetylcholine, histamine and prostaglandins, which increase the intensity of nociceptors to the effects of bradykinin.

Nociceptors (noxious sensation receptors) are specialized neurones found throughout the body, especially in the skin. They are classified according to the speed at which they conduct impulses. Speed of conduction is dependent on the diameter of the axon and whether it is myelinated. Large axons conduct faster than smaller axons. Myelin acts as an electrical insulator to enhance the speed of transmission. There are two types of nociceptor:

Table 2.1 Characteristics of nociceptors and associated fibres (developed from Park and Fulton, 1991; Tyrer, 1992)

Characteristic	Mechanoceptors	Polymodal nociceptors
Respond to	Strong pressure over a wide skin area Strong stimuli Sudden heat (>44°C)	Tissue damage caused by mechanical, chemical and thermal insult Chemical mediators formed/ released by damaged tissue
Associated fibres and characteristics of fibres	Aδ fibres: small myelinated, primary afferent neurones Transmit quickly (part of withdrawal reflex) 10–25 m/s Responsible for transmission of first, rapid pain	C fibres: unmyelinated, primary afferent neurones Transmit slowly 1 m/s Responsible for transmission of second, slow pain
Sensation perceived	Sharp, localized pricking pain	Prolonged, dull ache, poorly localized
Threshold characteristic	Constant threshold beneath which stimulus not perceived	Respond to a range of stimuli and to a variety of intensity
Sensitivity		Become increasingly sensitive to further stimulation after damage
Termination point in spinal cord	Lamina 1 in grey matter of spinal cord	Lamina 2 in substantia gelatinosa

mechanoceptors and polymodal nociceptors, which are responsible for transmission of different pain impulses and which have different characteristics (Table 2.1). Both the Aδ and C fibres terminate in the dorsal horn of the spinal cord. The Aδ fibres terminate in lamina 1 and the C fibres terminate in the substantia gelatinosa of lamina 2.

A neurone which travels from the nociceptor to the spinal cord is called a presynaptic neurone and it is the postsynaptic neurones which transmit impulses onwards to the brain. The main neurotransmitter responsible for the transmission of pain at the spinal cord level is substance P. Others include angiotensin II, 5 hydroxytryptamine (5-HT), noradrenaline, cholecystokinin (CKK), somatostatin, enkephalins and endorphins of endogenous opioid peptides. Substance P facilitates T cell transmission, which results in the gate opening and pain perception increasing. The enkephalins produce analgesia, euphoria and nausea as well as other effects. β-endorphins, produced in the pituitary gland during periods of intense arousal, may be responsible for dulling/negating perception of pain from some injuries.

The Aδ postsynaptic neurones cross from the dorsal horn of the spinal cord over the central canal and via the spinothalamic tract to the thalamus (the first structure in the brain to process nociceptive information). This route is mainly involved in sensory-discriminatory potential. Some Aδ fibres ascend via the spinoreticular tract. This route is concerned with the arousal–motivational aspects of the pain experience. The C fibres, which are more abundant, ascend to the thalamus or reticular formation via a series of short connecting neurones. Nociceptive impulses are then transmitted on to the limbic system, which is the area of the brain responsible for emotion. The majority of nociceptive fibres terminate in the cerebral cortex.

Gate control theory

This theory basically proposes that there is a 'gate' in the dorsal horn of the spinal cord. The degree to which the gate is open or closed affects the degree of pain perception. Gate control theory proposes that large fibre inputs tend to close the gate, that the gate can be opened by small fibre inputs and that the gate is additionally influenced by descending controls from the brain (Fig. 2.2). The gate can be affected by a variety of factors; these factors are of

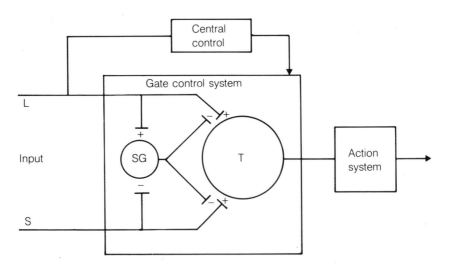

Figure 2.2 Gate control theory: L = large-diameter fibres; S = small-diameter fibres. The fibres project to the substantia gelatinosa (SG) and first central transmission (T) cells. The inhibitory effect exerted by SG on the afferent fibre terminals is increased by activity in L fibres and decreased by activity in S fibres. The central control trigger is represented by a line running from the large fibre system to the central control mechanisms; these mechanisms, in turn, project back to the gate control system. The T cells project to the action system. +, excitation; − inhibition. Reproduced from Melzack, R. and Wall, P.D. (1988) *The Challenge of Pain*, 2nd edn, by permission of the publishers Penguin Books.

clinical importance since if these gate-closing factors can be stimulated the child's perception of pain can be reduced or eliminated.

At the spinal cord level upward transmission of nociceptive impulses is dependent on the activation of the transmission cells (T) cells. T cell transmissions are inhibited by larger, myelinated fibres and facilitated by smaller, unmyelinated fibres. Additionally inhibition and facilitation are affected by the activity of the substantia gelatinosa (SG) cell. This cell is inhibited by the activity of C fibres and activated by large myelinated fibres responsible for touch and proprioception. The more active the SG cell the greater the inhibition of T cell transmission. Chemical inhibition can also occur via the release of γ-aminobutyric acid (GABA), which is released from cells in the dorsal lamina and which depolarizes the afferent terminals. This results in either inhibition or increased excitation.

Activity in Aδ and C nociceptive fibres has to outweigh the activity in the fibres responsible for touch and proprioception (which are also activated in injury and inflammation). Once activity has reached a critical level the transmission cell is 'tripped' and pain impulses can ascend to the brain, where pain perception occurs.

The theory therefore accounts for why 'rubbing something better' actually works – since the rubbing stimulates the large proprioception, pressure and touch fibres which can inhibit T cell transmission and reduce pain perception.

T cells can also be inhibited or facilitated by descending inhibition. If the child is relaxed the descending impulses can activate the SG cell and thus inhibit T cell transmission. However, if the child is tense and anxious then the child can experience a heightened perception of pain as a result of descending impulses from the limbic system which activate the T cells.

The descending inhibitory control system has an inhibitory effect on the T cell which is exerted by the brain stem. Additionally the distant noxious inhibitory control (DNIC) is thought to activate the descending inhibitory control system which, accounts for why intense stimulation at one site can inhibit stimulation at a distant site. The cognitive control mechanism triggers the cognitive processes to influence the gate control fibres.

Pain perception occurs through an an 'action system' and there is no such thing as a 'pain centre'. The immediate action on first perception of pain is warning and protection and a rapid assessment occurs of what has happened (Diamond and Coniam, 1991; McCaffery and Beebe, 1989; Melzack and Wall, 1988; Park and Fulton, 1991; Tyrer, 1992).

REFERENCES

Barasi, S. (1991) The physiology of pain. *Surgical Nurse*, **4**(5): 14–20.
Diamond, A.W. and Coniam, S.W. (1991) *The Management of Chronic Pain*. Oxford University Press, Oxford.

McCaffery, M. and Beebe, A. (1989) Pain: *Clinical Manual for Nursing Practice*. Mosby, St Louis.

Melzack, R. and Wall, P.D. (1965) Pain mechanisms: a new theory. *Science*, **150**: 971–979.

Melzack, R. and Wall, P.D. (1988) *The Challenge of Pain*, 2nd edn. Penguin Books, London.

Park, G. and Fulton, B. (1991) *The Management of Acute Pain*. Oxford University Press, Oxford.

Tyrer, S.P. (1992) Basic concepts of pain. In: Tyrer, S.P. (ed.) *Psychology, Psychiatry and Chronic Pain*. Butterworth Heinemann, Oxford.

Assessment and measurement of pain

INTRODUCTION

Effective pain management is fundamentally linked to the effective assessment of child's pain; without good pain assessment subsequent pain management strategies cannot be based on a good information base. Adult pain assessment is acknowledged to be problematic, with a number of studies demonstrating that nurses often inappropriately under-assess pain (Bondestam *et al.*, 1987; Dalton, 1989; Graffam, 1981; Seers, 1980). Bradshaw and Zeanah (1986) state that pain assessment is:

> One of the most common and most difficult tasks for nurses to accomplish (p. 315).

The difficulties faced in terms of the assessment of adult pain are compounded when concerned with assessing a child's pain. Children have a limited cognitive ability and limited verbal skills (Gaffney and Dunne, 1986; Bieri *et al.*, 1990), which makes understanding their pain difficult and creates difficulties for them in verbally expressing the quality and types of pain being experienced. However, studies show that even very young children are capable of describing their own pain (Ross and Ross, 1984), provided appropriate questions are asked. The situation is made more problematic by the relatively small amount of research-based literature available to turn to to provide reliable and valid assessment tools. Knowledge of many of the issues central to children's pain is also limited, although it must be acknowledged that this area is growing rapidly. Not only may the child have difficulties in communicating their experience to the nurse but there may be problems encountered in interpreting the information that the child is giving. Children also communicate their pain behaviourally and this is another area where professional knowledge is limited.

Pain is a plastic and complex experience and one which can only ever be measured and assessed indirectly. It is the result of these measurements and assessments that allows the nurse to draw conclusions about the child's experience of pain.

McGrath and Unruh (1987) draw attention to the two separate but linked issues to pain measurement and pain assessment and shows how each area requires further research. They state:

> Measurement refers to application of some metric to a specific element, usually intensity, of pain. Assessment is a much broader endeavor which encompasses the measurement of the interplay of different factors on the experience of pain . . . Whereas the measurement of pain in children is still in its early stages, research on the assessment of pediatric pain has not yet really begun. (p. 74)

The issue of pain measurement is crucial in terms of allowing appropriate intervention, evaluation and understanding of the child's pain. Assessment is vital if the health professional is to gain knowledge of the wider issues that the pain experience encompasses. A number of strategies exist that attempt to measure the intensity of pain.

Existing child pain assessment tools/methodologies have demonstrated the considerable methodological and developmental issues that complicate accurate and effective measurement (Thompson and Varni, 1986; McGrath, 1990).

Assessment of a child in pain requires an 'adequate and appropriate knowledge' base (Burr, 1987). This knowledge base needs to include an appreciation of the physical, cognitive, physiological and psychological stages of development of the child and an understanding of how a child may react to the stress of pain.

Three major approaches to pain assessment/measurement are commonly used: behavioural, psychological and physiological. These approaches arise from the three major components of pain: cognitive (or self-report); behavioural; and physiological (Table 3.1).

Although assessment of the child's pain can be made indirectly through the use of cognitive/self-report, behavioural and physiological approaches, no single approach can provide all the information required; as stated by Ross and Ross (1988):

> None of the components of the pain triad can stand on its own but . . .
> in combination with contextual factors they enable the nurses to draw
> some conclusions about the child's pain (p. 73).

Baker and Wong (1987) are cited in Whaley and Wong (1991) as developing QUESTT, which provides a model for pain assessment using both qualitative and quantitative techniques:

Table 3.1 Approaches to pain assessment

Self-report techniques
  Faces scales, Oucher, linear scales, visual analogue scales, simple descriptive scales
  Numeric scales, Poker Chip Tool, Eland Color Scale, Children's Global Rating Scale
  Pain questionnaires, pain diaries, pain interviews

Behavioural assessment
Infants:
  Cry, posture, facial expression, rigidity of torso, body movements
Children:
  Gauvain–Piquard Scale, Toddler–Preschooler Postoperative Pain Scale, CHEOPS

Physiological
  Cardiac, blood pressure, oxygenation, metabolic and endocrine changes

*Q*uestion the child
*U*se pain rating scales
*E*valuate behaviour and physiological changes
*S*ecure parents' involvement
*T*ake cause of pain into account
*T*ake action and evaluate results

This model provides a rich overview using a variety of strategies that should ensure that a holistic view of the child's pain, pain prevention and management result. Mathews *et al.* (1993) propose the use of the World Health Organization (WHO) model of the Consequences of Disease (WHO, 1980) as a basis for the use of a psychosocial model of pain assessment. The WHO classification system conceptualizes the consequences of disease occurring at:

four levels (planes of experience): (1) a disease itself;(2) an impairment (where the individual becomes aware of a symptom or abnormality); (3) a disability (or restriction in normal activity); and (4) a handicap (where the impairment or disability exerts an impact on normal social functioning).

Mathews *et al.* (1993) go on to explain how this model can be applied to children's pain:

As this model applies to pediatric pain, disease refers to the physical cause of pain (e.g., an incision), and an impairment is the pain itself. Inability to walk due to a painful incision would be considered a disability, as it restricts physical functioning. That disability might then become a handicap if it resulted in extended school absence and, consequently, restricted social interactions. However, these levels are not always easily distinguished, nor is there necessarily a causal, linear progression from one level to the next. (pp. 97–98)

The use of this model allows the health professional to consider and assess the impairing, disabling and handicapping factors and promotes active intervention in an attempt to decrease these effects. It provides an enhanced means of viewing not only the intensity of the pain but more importantly the consequence of the pain experience and it is worthy of careful consideration.

SELF-REPORT TECHNIQUES

Self-report techniques may sometimes be described as cognitive techniques. These measures rely on the child's ability to communicate their pain experience. They are based on the child's own description of their feelings and the images that they have of their pain. Self-reports (verbal, questionnaires and diaries) are important as they allow the nurse to collect and collate information about the quality, nature, duration and intensity of the pain. However, self-reports tend to be descriptive and qualitative rather than provide an objective measurement of the pain.

McGrath (1990) states that all cognitive measures of child pain have focused on the intensity rather than the qualities of the child's experience of pain. Due to younger children's limited language skills verbal reports are often seen to be unreliable (Eland and Anderson, 1977; Lynn, 1986). Additionally young children are often simply unable to understand what is being asked of them. Indeed, studies have shown that children under the age of 6 years rarely comprehend the word pain (Eland and Anderson, 1977). Mathews *et al.* (1993) suggest that the use of self-report measures has a lower age limit of 4 years. Tarbell *et al.* (1992) suggest that the scales that are available and applicable for older children:

cannot be used reliably with the prelingual child. (p. 273)

However, other recent research into the use of rating scales cited by Carpenter (1990) suggests that children as young as 5 years can competently utilize rating scales to report symptoms (Zelter *et al.*, 1988).

It should be borne in mind that children have differing levels of cognitive 'competence' in relation to their chronological age and the research studies do not (explicitly at least) appear to discuss the effects that illness and hospitalization may have in terms of creating some degree of regression. Additionally it must be acknowledged that pain rating tools which may be appropriate for older children will have less value in terms of the assessment of adolescents. One important factor that must also be considered when using pain assessment tools that are language oriented is that the child has a level of fluency in that language.

When choosing any self-report tool the nurse must also assess the child's age (or cognitive development) and abilities. It is also important to involve the child in the choice of tool so that they are working with an assessment tool that they understand and accept. Discussion of the pain assessment tool should also be considered proactively so that the child is introduced to the tool that they will be using before they are likely to experience the pain, where appropriate. This allows the child to familiarize themselves with it and ask any questions prior to the pain.

A variety of tools are available, including interviewing or questioning the child and their family, faces scales (Wong and Baker, 1988; Bieri *et al.*, 1990), the Oucher Scale (Beyer and Wells, 1989), the Poker Chip Tool (Hester, 1979), visual analogue scales and pain diaries (McCaffery and Beebe, 1989), the Eland Color Scale (Eland 1981, 1985) and the Children's Global Rating Scale (Carpenter, 1990).

Carpenter (1990) reports that lack of cognitive and linguistic ability limits the appropriateness of many self-report measures since young children are unable to self-evaluate and complete such tools.

Rating scales provide basic quantitative data on the intensity of the pain experience. Three main divisions occur: category rating scales (words, faces, poker chips); visual analogue scales; and graded thermometers. These scales rely on the child choosing a point on the scale that matches their own pain. This at first glance seems appropriate, although McGrath (1989) states that:

> it is important to recognize that the numerical values associated with different intensity levels in these scales are often selected by adults, so that the numbers do not necessarily reflect a child's own perception of pain intensity. (p. 205)

Although self-report tools are a valuable means of generating information on the child's pain they can be distorted by the child's reluctance to discuss their pain for fear of the consequences (Eland, 1981; McCaffery, 1972; Gross and Gardner, 1980). Health care professionals should therefore be guided by the principle that pain should be assumed to be present unless there is real evidence for its absence. The Pain Management Guidelines Panel (1992) has as its first guideline for the effective management of acute pain that:

> children often cannot or will not report pain to their health care providers. Thus, health-care professionals should have a high degree of suspicion of pain. (p. 230)

Faces scales

A variety of faces scales have been developed in an attempt to allow assessment of the younger child who does not have well-developed verbal and/or reading skills. The scales vary from cartoon-type faces to more realistic drawings of a face displaying characteristic pain features. Most, but not all of the scales, show tears on the face representing the most hurt or pain. Generally these tools have been well evaluated and are helpful in assessing young children's pain. However, criticism from Carpenter (1990) about the use of face-type scales is representative of some of the concerns that have been voiced. Carpenter (1990) suggests the major concerns:

(a) children's level of cognitive development may influence their ratings, and (b) they exert little control over the psychologic construct being measured. (p. 234)

He illustrates this point by recalling an example of a 6-year-old boy who used a face-type scale in a concrete fashion. This boy who was using the scale in assessing the pain experienced in relation to a medical procedure chose a face showing a low level of distress, stating that 'I get real scared, but I don't cry.' Perhaps this literal use of faces scales by some children needs to be carefully considered by nurses using this type of scale. Careful explanation of what the drawings or cartoons represent is obviously of paramount importance.

Perhaps the most widely recognized faces scale is the **Wong and Baker Faces Rating Scale** (1988) (Fig. 3.1), which has been shown to be the most preferred scale by children aged 3–18 years when compared to other assessment scales used. The Wong and Baker scale uses six faces numbered 0–5 to measure pain affect, with the faces varying from a smiling face through to neutral and to total misery. The sixth face is crying. This cartoon-based tool is often seen to be appealing to the child, who may readily relate to the cartoons.

Douhit (1990) describes the Faces Rating Scale as being the optimal scale for use on children aged 3–7 years. **Douhit's Faces Rating Scale** (Fig. 3.2) is based on five cartoon faces running from a happy, smiling face on the left to an obviously miserable face on the right. The fourth and fifth faces are crying. The faces are a little more detailed than the Wong and Baker Faces Scale. There is little published evidence to suggest that this scale is more reliable or valid than Wong and Baker.

Figure 3.1 Wong and Baker Faces Scale

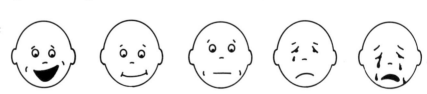

Figure 3.2 Douhit's Faces Scale.

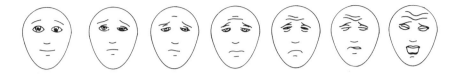

Figure 3.3 The Faces Pain Scale. (Reproduced with permission from Bieri *et al.*, *Pain*, **41**: 139–150; published by Elsevier Science Publishers BV, 1990).

Bieri *et al.* (1990) propose that the **Faces Pain Scale** (Fig. 3.3) developed as a result of their study has 'superior scaling properties' and:

> does not confuse the pain severity dimension with a happiness dimension, evident in several other scales. (p. 147)

This scale was derived through a phased piece of research from children's drawings of pain. The scale consists of seven faces that again show pain affect from a relaxed face on the left and a face showing intense pain on the right. None of the faces have tears so this is less likely to get confused with unhappiness and sadness.

Bieri *et al.* (1990) also report that 6–8-year-olds had a clear understanding of the term pain and what is meant by different levels of intensity of pain. Children principally used the eyes and mouth to display facial changes in pain reaction in their drawings. This scale has been reported to have been used successfully on 3-year-old children.

Oucher

The Oucher (Beyer, 1984) was developed from the faces scale using six photographs (Fig. 3.4) arranged on a vertical scale aligned to a vertical numerical scale marked in intervals of 20 (0–100). The numerical scale runs 0 = 'no hurt', 1–29 'little hurts', 30–69 'middle hurts', 70–99 'big hurts', and 100 'biggest hurt you could ever have'. The child is able to choose any number between 0 and 100, not just those on the Oucher. The scale aims to measure the report of pain intensity in children aged 3–12 years.

Studies have suggested that the Oucher has content validity (Beyer and Arandine, 1986; Arandine *et al.*, 1988). The photographic scale runs from a non-pain face to a most-pain face using a 3-year-old male child. Ross and Ross (1988) report the Oucher to be useful for young children and those with language difficulties. Arandine *et al.* (1988) propose that children as young as 3 years old can use the Oucher scale to report intensity of pain. Beyer *et al.* (1992) report the development of an ethnic version of the Oucher and the reassessment of the poster in terms of overall design, ethnicity and gender.

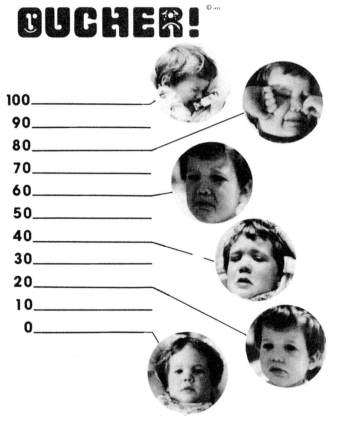

Figure 3.4 The Oucher. (Reproduced by permission of Judith E. Beyer, RN, PhD, copyright 1983).

LINEAR SCALES

These scales are mostly based on a horizontal line with a mark at one end indicating no pain and a mark at the other end indicating worst/extreme pain. Some scales are represented vertically.

Visual Analogue Scale

This is a horizontal line, usually about 10 cm long, that has end points marked 'no pain' and 'worst pain' (Fig. 3.5). It may be possible to adapt the end point markings to suit the child so that it reflects their own feeling about their pain, for example 'great' and 'really yucky', although this aspect does not appear to have been researched. The Visual Analogue Scale (VAS) allows

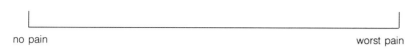

no pain   worst pain

Figure 3.5 Visual Analogue Scale for Pain Intensity (with end markings).

biggest hurt

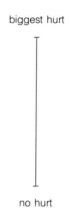

no hurt

Figure 3.6 Simple pain thermometer.

the child absolute freedom over where they place their mark on the line to reflect the intensity of their pain. The pain score is derived by measuring along the line from the no-pain marker to the child's mark and recording that measurement. Ross and Ross (1988) suggest that the relative lack of markings results in this being very appropriate for children with limited vocabularies or language skills.

Some research (Beyer and Arandine, 1986) suggests that a vertical line using end markers of 'no hurt' and 'biggest hurt' may be conceptually easier for children to handle and they describe this as a pain thermometer (Fig. 3.6). Szyfelbein *et al.* (1985) demonstrated that children undergoing painful burns dressings found that the pain thermometer was the children's choice as the best way of expressing their pain.

Simple descriptive scales

Simple descriptive scales are based on the VAS and generally provide a reliable means of measuring pain. They can be used by children aged 5 years and older (Fig. 3.7). These scales have slash marks placed at regular intervals, with words that help the child to decide what part of the scale best describes their pain. The descriptions that accompany the scale can vary according to the scale. Normally the numbers run from 0 to 5 or 0 to 10 (Whaley and Wong, 1991).

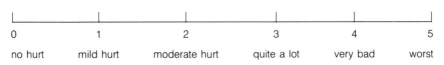

Figure 3.7 Simple descriptive scale.

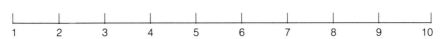

Figure 3.8 Numerical scale.

Numerical scales

A numerical scale runs along a horizontal line with regular marks along it (0–10 etc.) with 0 representing no pain and the upper number representing worst pain (Fig. 3.8).

Poker Chip Tool (Hester, 1979)

This tool was developed to allow children to rate their pain 'concretely' by using chips that are described as being 'pieces of hurt'. The child is able to choose the number of poker chips that best describe how much they hurt. Originally all four poker chips were white; however, Molsberry (1979) (cited in Wong and Baker, 1988) used five poker chips (four red ones for pain and one white one representing no pain). The more chips that the child chooses the worse their hurt. Although Hester provides some evidence of concurrent validity by demonstrating that Poker Chip Tool scores correlated well with children's behavioural and verbal responses to an immunization injection, Ross and Ross (1988) question issues central to its validity. They suggest that young children may not have mastered number concepts, which would make its use questionable. However, they propose that making the poker chips obviously different sizes would be an appropriate modification.

Eland Color Scale (Eland, 1981, 1985, 1988)

One of the most important aspects of this scale is that it not only provides information on the child's level of pain but just as importantly the location(s) of their pain (Fig. 3.9). The scale provides an outline figure (front and back view) with four boxes (no pain/hurt to worst pain/hurt) for the child to colour in with their choice of colour. Eland suggests that eight crayons (yellow, orange, red, green, blue, purple, brown and black) are presented to the child, who is allowed to choose which colour most accurately represents the levels

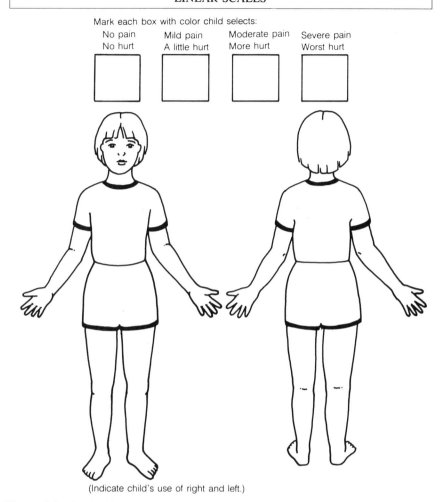

Figure 3.9 Eland Color Scale.

of their pain. Once the 'key' has been created the child is then encouraged to colour in the outlines where they hurt using the colour that is appropriate. The child is encouraged to locate the drawing in respect to time. Researchers have found that black and red are the most frequently chosen colours used to portray pain (Unruh *et al.*, 1983; Kurylyszn *et al.*, 1987).

Children's Global Rating Scale (Carpenter, 1990)

The Children's Global Rating Scale (CGRS) allows children to rate their pain against a set of five lines (0–4) (Fig. 3.10). Line 0 is straight and the lines become progressively wavier, with line 4 being the waviest. The rationale behind the choice of this approach is that the lines (or stimuli) are based on

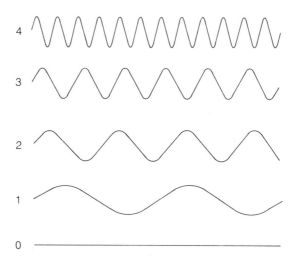

Figure 3.10 Children's Global Rating Scale.

the way that pain is 'commonly characterized or represented in children's books and and comics' and has neutral properties when compared with other tools such as faces scales. Carpenter's study suggests that the CGRS has scope for objectively and validly measuring young children's pain. This scale was used on children as young as 4 years old. Further research needs to be undertaken to test its validity and reliability.

Pain questionnaires

A variety of assessment tools are available that fall into this category: Varni–Thompson Pediatric Pain Questionnaire (Varni *et al.*, 1987); Adolescent Paediatric Pain Tool (Savedra *et al.*, 1993); and the McGill Pain Questionnaire, which is mostly used with adult patients (Melzack, 1975).

Generally these questionnaires allow a wide range of data to be collected rather than simply focusing on the intensity of pain.

The **Pediatric Pain Questionnaire** (PPQ) (Varni *et al.*, 1987) has three components: a child, an adolescent and a parent form. It was originally developed for chronic pain assessment in children and it collects information on the sensory, affective and evaluative components (through a pain word list) of the pain experience, pain location and intensity (by using a body outline and a visual analogue scale). Comprehensive assessment tools such as this provide a firm basis from which to manage the child's subsequent care.

Savedra *et al.* (1993) developed the **Adolescent Pediatric Pain Tool** (APPT), a multidimensional tool that assesses three dimensions of pain: location, intensity and quality. It was designed for children aged 8–17 with multiethnic backgrounds. It comprises a body outline with a segmented overlay (front and back), a word graphic rating scale and a 56-word pain descriptor list (grouped in sensory, affective and evaluative qualities). The descriptor list was derived from studies on children's own choices. Initial findings suggest that the APPT 'consistently documented the location, intensity and quality of postoperative pain experiences over time'.

Diaries

These provide a useful way of allowing the child to explore their pain experience and to document pain episodes. They also demonstrate the range of experiences that the child may report as being in some way painful (McGrath, 1989). They also allow the child to report the multidimensional nature of the pain experience (social, emotional etc.) as it affects them.

Pain interviews

Although simply asking the child about their pain may seem the most obvious means of finding out about it, care needs to be taken in phrasing the questions, who is asking the questions and the context of the questions. Questioning the child is open to bias and misinterpretation and rarely leads to a quantifiable measurable response. The major issue to consider is the child's understanding of the outcome of their response. If they anticipate an injection when they say that they have 'awful pain' they may simply report less pain to avoid the injection. McGrath (1989) proposed the use of generated and supplied format questions to gain a comprehensive interview and this area needs further research.

The language of pain used by children and adolescents has also undergone study. Wilkie *et al.* (1990) have developed a 56-word list that is reported to be relatively free of gender, ethnic or developmental biases. Jerett and Evans (1986) also found that children used different words when describing pain compared to the word list already established by the McGill Pain Questionnaire. Words used by children in the 5 years to 6 years 11 months group includes 'bullet', 'upset' and 'yucky' and although there were some similarities between that group and the children aged 7 years to 9 years 6 months additional words were used, including 'dizzy', 'disappointed' and 'weird'.

BEHAVIOURAL ASSESSMENT

Two basic categories become clear within behavioural assessment: infants and children. With both infants and children behavioural assessment allows assumptions to be drawn about what the behaviour is representing. However, it is often difficult to distinguish pain-related behaviour from behaviour resulting from other causes of distress, especially in the infant group. Behavioural techniques do not actively involve the child and therefore issues such as cognitive ability and linguistic skill are not problematic. The range of behaviours measured include cry, posture, facial expression, rigidity of the torso and body movements. However, none of these is definitely indicative of pain – rather they are suggestive of pain. Other behaviours exhibited by the child or infant include withdrawing socially, decreasing their activities and developing poor sleep patterns, and they may experience mood changes.

Behavioural assessment is unobtrusive, non-invasive and does not place any demands on the child or infant. On the other hand, it places considerable demands on the nurse who is assessing and interpreting those behaviours. McGrath (1990) states:

> Children's behaviors are not simple and direct expressions of the quality or intensity of their pains. (p. 44)

This is also supported by the work of LeBaron and Zeltzer (1984). Children's behaviours may reflect learnt coping mechanisms and will ultimately reflect their usual methods of expressing pain. Criterion-based behavioural assessment has been the focus of recent studies and it is only recently that the sophistication and range of response that children have to pain experiences have been noted (Van der Does, 1989).

Considering the 'risks' associated with interpreting, or rather misinterpreting, a child's pain behaviour in respect to their actual experience, it is worrying to note that when there is a discrepancy between the observer's assessment and the child's own report studies would suggest that it is the child who is not believed (Moinpour *et al.*, 1990).

BEHAVIOURAL ASSESSMENT: INFANTS

Grunau and Craig (1987) state that neonatal pain behaviour:

> occurs prior to the possibility of learned reaction patterns. Thus it forms the basis for subsequent maturation and integration of sensory, cognitive, affective, and behavioral events, within specific familial and cultural contexts, which may mediate the experience and behavioral responses to noxious stimuli in children and adults. (pp. 395–396)

Although infant behaviour is an area that has attracted a reasonable amount of attention it is still under-researched and the assessments have not been standardized (Carter, 1993). Porter (1989) suggests that:

> Behavioural measures are often not applicable to premature or sick infants who, owing to their immaturity, clinical conditions, or therapeutic programs simply do not demonstrate behavioral responses to

pain ... behavioral assessments ... reflect the subjective judgement
of observers rather than the infants' individualized response to pain.
(p. 553)

Facial expression

Neonatal facial pain studies have developed from work performed by
Darwin (1872) and subsequently Izard (1971), who demonstrated that facial
expressions are universal in meaning. Neonatal expressions which appear to
be associated with pain seem to be universal in meaning and a fairly
sophisticated method of communicating pain. Work by Craig *et al.* (1992)
reports that neonatal facial expression of pain is similar to adult expression
of pain. However, Grunau *et al.* (1990) state:

it is not as yet clear whether a constrained set of facial actions is pain
specific. (pp. 295–296)

Facial expression is measured by tools such as the Neonatal Facial Coding
System (NFCS) (Grunau and Craig, 1990) or the Facial Action Coding System
(FACS) (Ekman and Friesen, 1978). Izard *et al.* (1980) demonstrated that
facial pain expression is characterized by closed eyes and an angular squarish
mouth, whereas Grunau and Craig (1987) found that the most significant
responses were vertical stretch mouth and taut tongue:

Taut tongue in combination with the facial grimace cluster of actions
may signify greater pain sensitivity or expressivity ...
... rapid facial grimaces consisting of lowered brows, eyes squeezed
shut, deepening of the naso-labial furrow and open lips. (Grunau *et al.*,
1990, p. 303)

Grunau *et al.* (1990) also found that a cupped tongue was a possible
indicator of pain in neonates. Interestingly, tongue protrusion was never
seen in response to the painful stimuli, which was an injection of vitamin
K. Grunau and Craig (1987) found an immense variety of differences within
the acknowledged pain expression which was indicative of the degree of
handling, stress and pain. Johnston *et al.* (1993) found that in response to
sharp, acute pain infants (aged 32 weeks gestation to 4 months) demonstrated a characteristic expression with open lips, mouth stretch, taut
tongue, and naso-labial furrow with brow bulge and eye squeeze. Interestingly the premature infants demonstrated an increased incidence of horizontal
mouth stretch. Craig *et al.* (1993) report greater facial activity in the
full-term infants in the study than in the preterm infants, which is supportive
of Johnston *et al.*'s (1993) findings.

Overall studies have found that facial expression is the most consistent
element in the neonate's response to pain (Craig *et al.*, 1993; Dale, 1986,
1989; Marvin and Pomietto, 1991).

Cry

Infant cry is the most frequently studied factor associated with infant pain. Grunau et al. (1990) state:

> Cry is a probabilistic sign of pain, but pain may occur without cry, and cry occurs in response to non painful events. (p. 303)

Owens and Todt (1984) demonstrated that in response to a heel stab 2-day-old babies consistently and immediately cried and they go on to state:

> It makes sense that crying would begin very quickly if it is to communicate to care givers the potential of continuing tissue damage. (p. 84)

Cries tend to vary in their duration and intensity, seemingly in response to the duration and intensity of the stimulus (Wasz-Hockert et al., 1968). Owens (1986) reports that although pain cries are not qualitatively different from other cries, the intensity of the cry is significant in respect to both the context in which it occurs and the motivation of the person hearing the cry.

Wolff (1974), however, suggests that different cries have different functions and that the hunger, anger and pain cries elicit different responses, with the pain cry eliciting an urgent need to respond to it and act upon it. The cry which is recognized as the pain cry can be easily recognized by people other than the primary care giver and training can increase the responsiveness of the listener. Levine and Gordon (1982) showed that pain cries were not modified by cultural background, age or social rearing practices. Grunau and Craig (1987) showed that boys cried sooner than girls to a stimulus.

Owens and Todt (1984) demonstrated that healthy term babies cried for approximately 207 seconds after heel stab. Porter et al. (1986) in a study on neonatal cry during circumcision suggest that an infant's cries are perceived by adult listeners as having differing degrees of urgency, with an increase in the intensity of the noxious stimulus creating more urgent cries. Porter et al. (1986) found that the pain cry had distinctive properties, including longer bouts of crying with short bouts of quiet with distinctive fundamental frequencies. Fuller (1990) also notes that the characteristics of cry change during different phases of circumcision. Johnston et al. (1993) found that preterm infants' cries were characteristically more alerting to their care givers as they had a higher fundamental frequency.

Body movements

This is another area that has been studied although no specific motor response has been shown to be characteristic of pain. Franck (1986) suggests that an objective assessment tool could be based on the intensity, number and velocity of leg movements. Cote et al. (1991) indicate (from a small ethological study) that acute distress is evidenced behaviourally by both legs moving (along with frowning and crying). In Cote's pilot study she notes that the 'feet of the infant were more expressive than the fingers'. Porter (1989) reports that newborns can actively and precisely avoid pain. One of the problems with using body movements as a form of assessment is that it may not be appropriate to use with the very small preterm babies who are physically constrained within high-tech hospital environments. Craig *et al.* (1993) report that again body movements/gross motor activity is not very specific in terms of a characteristic response although the full-term infants were more active than the preterm infants in the study.

BEHAVIOURAL ASSESSMENT: CHILDREN

A number of observational tools exist to allow the nurse to assess the child's pain behaviours. These have been developed in an attempt to reliably assess young children's pain (1–5 years) who are unable or less able to use the self-report measures previously discussed. They aim to provide a useful assessment for the clinical setting. The currently available behavioural assessment tools reflect the purpose for which they were developed. Gauvain-Piquard *et al.* (1987, 1991) are developing an observational scale for children with cancer aged 2–6 years. This is based on 15 behaviours which are subdivided into pain behaviours, anxiety behaviours and psychomotor alterations.

Tarbell *et al.* (1992) report the development of the **Toddler–Preschooler Postoperative Pain Scale** (TPPPS), which has been devised for use in children aged 1–5 years. The TPPPS is composed of seven items that are divided into three observational categories: vocal pain expression, facial pain expression and bodily pain expression. These items were derived from previous studies involving observed postoperative pain behaviours. Tarbell *et al.* report that the tool is suitable for clinical use.

- *Vocal pain expression*: verbal pain complaint/cry; scream; groan; moan; grunt
- *Facial pain expression*: open mouth; lips pulled back at corners; squint; closed eyes; furrow forehead; brow bulge
- *Bodily pain expression*: restless motor behaviour; rub or touch painful area

Another tool devised for the assessment of postoperative pain is the **Children's Hospital of Eastern Ontario Pain Scale (CHEOPS)** (Table 3.2), which is based in six categories of pain-related behaviours and developed by McGrath *et al.* (1985).

The pain behaviour categories are: crying; facial expression; verbalization (both pain and non-pain related); movement of the torso; tactile activity; and leg movements. Pain behaviours are scored and the score will indicate pain. McGrath (1989) suggests that although CHEOPS is a good tool for

Table 3.2 Behavioural definitions and scoring of CHEOPS

Item	Behaviour	Score	Definition
Cry	No cry	1	Child is not crying
	Moaning	2	Child is moaning or quietly vocalizing; silent cry
	Crying	2	Child is crying, but the cry is gentle or whimpering
	Scream	3	Child is in a full-lunged cry; sobbing: may be scored with complaint or without complaint
Facial	Composed	1	Neutral facial expression
	Grimace	2	Score only if definite negative facial expression
	Smiling	0	Score only if definite positive facial expression
Child verbal	None	1	Child not talking
	Other complaints	1	Child complains, but not about pain: e.g. 'I want to see mommy' or 'I am thirsty'
	Pain complaints	2	Child complains about pain
	Both complaints	2	Child complains about pain and about other things; e.g., 'It hurts; I want mommy'
	Positive	0	Child makes any positive statement or talks about other things without complaint
Torso	Neutral	1	Body (not limbs) is at rest; torso is inactive
	Shifting	2	Body is in motion in a shifting or serpentine fashion
	Tense	2	Body is arched or rigid
	Shivering	2	Body is shuddering or shaking involuntarily
	Upright	2	Child is in vertical or upright position
	Restrained	2	Body is restrained
Touch	Not touching	1	Child is not touching or grabbing at wound
	Reach	2	Child is reaching for but not touching wound
	Touch	2	Child is gently touching wound or wound area
	Grab	2	Child is grabbing vigorously at wound
	Restrained	2	Child's arms are restrained
Legs	Neutral	1	Legs may be in any position but are relaxed; includes gentle swimming or serpentine-like movements
	Squirming/kicking	2	Definitive uneasy or restless movements in the legs and/or striking out with foot or feet
	Drawn up/tensed	2	Legs tensed and/or pulled up tightly to body and kept there
	Standing	2	Standing, crouching or kneeling
	Restrained	2	Child's legs are being held down

assessing distress, it 'has not been demonstrated to be a pure pain measure' (p. 203). However, in a study by Tyler *et al.* (1993) CHEOPS was seen to be a valid measurement tool when compared with observational pain scales and visual analogue and a faces scale (within the limitations of the measurement techniques used).

Pain behaviour assessment of children should be used cautiously since many factors can influence the child's behaviour, such as the presence of their parent, the relative stressfulness of a situation and their own previously developed coping strategies. Additionally medication and the child's condition are influences that must be taken into consideration.

PHYSIOLOGICAL MEASURES OF PAIN

A level of debate occurs about the usefulness of and reliability of physiological measurements of pain. The parameters that are measured include heart rate, blood pressure, respiratory rate, oxygenation changes, and endocrine and metabolic responses. The difficulty is partly due to the fact that it is problematic determining if the physiological changes result from the pain or from other stressors. However, Ross and Ross (1988) suggest that:

> the potential value of the physiological indices of pain is inversely related to age, with their greatest utility occurring in infancy as an adjunct to behavioral observation. (p. 85).

One area that bears greater investigation relates to the relationship between β-endorphin plasma levels and pain reports (Szyfelbein *et al.*, 1985). It should also be noted that prolonged pain leads to adaptation, which may result in pain not presenting through physiological assessment (McCaffery, 1977).

Physiological indices are an area that have greater significance with infant pain assessment than child assessment, even though most studies relate physiological changes to the acute short pain of heel stab or the longer acute pain of circumcision. Critics of physiological assessment suggest that neither of these situations satisfactorily mimics the pains that the sick neonate is likely to experience. Additionally Craig *et al.* (1993) suggest that physiological indices may not be the most useful measure of an infant's pain owing to the inconsistency in response. The infant's physiological indices did not, apart from oxygen saturation, differentiate between the swab and the lance. Cardiac response has been investigated as it is the easiest non-invasive physiological parameter to measure. Owens and Todt (1984), Beaver (1987) and Williamson and Williamson (1988) have all shown that a painful stimulus evokes a bidirectional cardiac response, that is, an immediate elevation of heart rate. Owens and Todt (1984) investigating the neonate's response to a heel stab showed that a mean rise of 44 beats per minute (bpm) to an average of 179 bpm occurred and it took an average of 3.5 minutes to return to pre-procedure baseline.

The work related to blood pressure response is less convincing, although the weight of evidence suggests that blood pressure is initially increased as a result of a noxious stimulus but that it returns to baseline faster than heart rate (Beaver, 1987).

Williamson and Williamson (1983) in a study on response to circumcision showed that transcutaneous oxygen levels demonstrated an initial appreciable drop, with a delay in recovery and often a labile period after the stimulus. Beaver (1987) demonstrated in respect to a heel stab an appreciable drop in transcutaneous oxygen tension ($tcpO_2$) readings within 5 seconds of receiving the stimulus, with the readings continuing to drop until 65 seconds after the stimulus and showing only slight recovery 95 seconds post stimulus. Brown (1987) reports on an initial slight rise that was followed by a further rise after completion of the procedure. Rawlings et al. (1980) suggest that changes in $tcpO_2$ measurement are reflective of the effects of crying which causes either a decrease in alveolar ventilation or a secondary increase in intrathoracic pressure due to a right-to-left shunt. Rawlings et al. (1980) showed that respiratory rate during circumcision was increased by 7–10 breaths per minute compared to baseline criteria.

Harpin and Rutter (1982) in a study of 124 infants (25–40 weeks gestation) examined palmar sweating in response to heel stab. Infants less than 37 weeks gestation demonstrated a 200–300% increase in palmar water loss within a minute of heel stab. This palmar water loss became more pronounced as the infants became older.

Evidence now supports the neonate's capability of showing endocrine changes in response to painful stimuli. Anand et al. (1985) demonstrated a severe catabolic reaction to surgery with increases in glycerol, adrenaline and noradrenaline plasma levels. Increases in plasma cortisol levels (intra and post procedure) have been noted in neonates undergoing circumcision without anaesthesia (Gunnar et al., 1981).

However, very few comprehensive neonatal assessment tools have been assessed within the clinical setting exist and at present this is an area that needs further development. Porter (1993) reports PAIN (Pain Assessment Inventory for Neonates), which is used for assessing acute pain but which still needs further clinical trials. Sparshott (1989) has developed a chart for recording pain responses in the neonate which appears to be developed from established literature. However, no evidence is presented to suggest its construct validity or reliability. Attia et al. (1987) propose a clinical scoring system that measures the effectiveness of analgesia administered postoperatively. This is based on a pain score derived from the 10 scoring criteria: sleep; facial expression; quality of cry; spontaneous motor activity; spontaneous excitability and responsiveness to ambient stimulation; constant and excessive flexion of fingers and toes; suckling;

sucking; global evaluation of tone; consolability; and sociabilty. However, again it is not possible to assess its construct validity.

REFERENCES

Anand, K.J.S., Brown, M.J. and Causon, R.C. (1985) Can the human neonate mount an endocrine response and metabolic response to surgery? *Journal of Pediatric Surgery*, **20**: 41–48.

Arandine, C.R., Beyer, J.E. and Tompkins, J.M. (1988) Children's pain perception before and after analgesia: a study of instrument construct validity and related issues. *Journal of Pediatric Nursing*, **3**(1): 11–23.

Attia, J., Amiel-Timson, C., Mayer, M.-N., Shnider, S.M. and Barrier, G. (1987) Measurement of post operative pain and narcotic administration in infants using a new clinical scoring system. *Anesthesiology*, **67**(3A): A532.

Baker, C. and Wong, D. (1987) Q.U.E.S.T.T.: a process of pain assesssment in children. *Orthopedic Nursing*, **6**(1): 11–21.

Beaver, P.K. (1987) Premature infants' response to touch and pain: can nurses make a difference? *Neonatal Network*, **6**(3): 13–17.

Beyer, J.E. (1984) *The Oucher: A User's Manual and Technical Report*. Hospital Play Equipment Co., Evanston, IL.

Beyer, J.E. and Arandine, C.R. (1986) Content validity of an instrument to measure young children's perceptions of the intensity of their pain. *Journal of Pediatric Nursing*, **1**: 386–395.

Beyer, J.E. and Wells, N. (1989) The assessment of pain in children. *Pediatric Clinics of North America*, **36**(4): 837–854.

Beyer, J.E., Deynes, M.J. and Villareu, A.M. (1992) The creation, validation and continuing development of the Oucher: a measure of pain intensity in children. *Journal of Pediatric Nursing: Nursing Care of Children and Families*, **7**(5): 335–346.

Bieri, D., Reeve, R.A., Champion, G.D., Addicoat, L. and Ziegler, J.B. (1990) The faces pain scale for the self-assessment of the severity of pain experienced by children: development, initial validation, and preliminary investigation for ratio scale properties. *Pain*, **41**: 139–150.

Bondestam, E., Hovgren, K., Johansson, F.G., Jern, S., Herlitz, J. and Holmberg, S. (1987) Pain assessment by patients and nurses in the early phase of acute myocardial infarction. *Journal of Advanced Nursing*, **12**(6): 677–682.

Bradshaw, C. and Zeanah, P.D. (1986) Pediatric nurses' assessments of pain in children. *Journal of Pediatric Nursing*, **1**: 314–322.

Brown, L. (1987) Physiological responses to cutaneous pain in neonates. *Neonatal Network*, **6**(3): 18–22.

Burr, S. (1987) Pain in childhood. *Nursing*, **24**: 890–896.

Carpenter, P.J. (1990) New method for measuring young children's self-report of fear and pain. *Journal of Pain and Symptom Management*, **5**(4): 233–240.

Carter, B. (1993) Care of the child in pain. In: Carter, B. (ed), *Manual of Paediatric Intensive Care Nursing*. Chapman & Hall, London, pp. 280–291.

Cote, J.J., Morse, J.M. and James, S.G. (1991) The pain response of the postoperative newborn. *Journal of Advanced Nursing*, **16**: 378–387.

Craig, K.D., Prkachin, K.M. and Grunau, R.V.E. (1992) The facial expression of pain. In: Turk, D.C. and Melzack, R. (eds), *The Handbook of Pain Assessment.* Guilford, New York, pp. 257–276.

Craig, K.D., Whitfield, M.F., Grunau, R.V.E., Linton, J. and Hadjistavropouos, H.D. (1993) Pain in the preterm neonate: behavioural and physiological indices. *Pain,* 52: 287–299.

Dale, J.C. (1986) A multidimensional study of infants' responses to painful stimuli. *Pediatric Nursing,* 12: 27–31.

Dale, J.C. (1989) A multidimensional study of infant behavior associated with assumed painful stimuli: phase II. *Journal of Pediatric Health Care,* 3: 34–38.

Dalton, J.A. (1989) Nurses' perceptions of their pain assessment skill, pain management practices and attitudes towards pain. *Oncology Nursing Forum,* 16(62): 225–21.

Darwin, C. (1872) *The Expression of the Emotions of Man and Animals.* John Murray, London.

Douhit, J.L. (1990) Psychosocial assessment and management of pediatric pain. *Journal of Emergency Nursing,* 16(3) part 1: 168–170.

Ekman, P. and Friesen, W.V. (1978) *The Facial Action Coding System (FACS).* Consulting Psychologists Press, Palo Alto, CA.

Eland, J. (1981) Minimizing pain associated with prekindergarten intramuscular injections. *Issues in Comprehensive Pediatric Nursing,* 5: 361–372.

Eland, J.M. (1985) The child who is hurting. *Seminars in Oncology Nursing,* 1: 116–122.

Eland, J.M. (1988) Persistence of pain research: one nurse researcher's efforts. *Recent Advances in Nursing*; 21: 43–62.

Eland, J.M. and Anderson, J.E. (1977) The experience of pain in children. In: Jacox, A.K. (ed.), *Pain: A Source Book for Nurses and Other Health Professionals.* Little, Brown & Co., Boston, pp. 453–473.

Franck, L.S. (1986) A new method to quantitatively describe pain behavior in infants. *Nursing Research,* 35(1): 28–31.

Fuller, B.F. (1990) Potential acoustic measures of infant pain and arousal. In: Turk, D.C. and Melzack, R. (eds), *The Handbook of Pain Assessment.* Guilford, New York, pp. 137–145.

Gaffney, A. and Dunne, G. (1986) Developmental aspects of children's definitions of pain. *Pain,* 26: 105–117.

Gauvain-Piquard, A., Rodery, C., Rezvani, A. and Lemerle, J. (1987) Pain in children aged 2–6 years: a new observational rating scale elaborated in a pediatric oncology unit. Preliminary report. *Pain,* 31: 177–188.

Gauvain-Piquard, A., Rodery, C., Francois, P. *et al.* (1991) Validity assessment of DEGR[R] scale for observational rating of 2–6 year old child pain. *Journal of Pain and Symptom Management,* 6(Abstract): 171.

Graffam, S. (1981) Congruence of nurse–patient expectations regarding nursing intervention in pain. *Nursing Leadership,* 4(2): 120–125.

Gross, S. and Gardner, G. (1980) Child pain: treatment approaches. In: Smith, W., Merskey, H. and Gross, S. (eds), *Pain: Meaning and Management.* SP Medical and Scientific Books, New York.

Grunau, R.V.E. and Craig, K.D. (1987) Pain expression in neonates: facial action and cry. *Pain,* 28(3): 395–410.

Grunau, R.V.E. and Craig, K.D. (1990) Facial activity as a measure of neonatal pain expression. In: Tyler, D.C. and Krane, E.J. (eds), *Advances in Pain Research and Therapy*, Vol. 15, *Pediatric Pain*. Raven Press, New York.

Grunau, R.V.E., Johnston, C.C. and Craig, K.D. (1990) Neonatal facial and cry responses to invasive and non-invasive procedures. *Pain*, **42**: 293–305.

Gunnar, M.R., Fisch, R.O., Korsvik, S. and Donhowe, J.M. (1981) The effects of circumcision on serum cortisol and behavior. *Psychoneuroendocrinology*, **6**: 269–275.

Harpin, V.A. and Rutter, N. (1982) Development of emotional sweating in the newborn infant. *Archives of Disease in Childhood*, **57**: 691.

Hester, N. (1979) The preoperational child's reaction to immunization. *Nursing Research*, **28**: 250–255.

Izard, C.E. (1971) *The Face of Emotion*. Appleton-Century Crofts, New York.

Izard, C.E., Huebner, R.R., Resser, D., McGiness, G.C. and Dougherty, L.M. (1980) The infant's ability to produce discrete emotional expressions. *Developmental Psychology*, **16**: 132–140.

Jerrett, M.D. and Evans, K. (1986) Children's pain vocabulary. *Journal of Advanced Nursing*, **11**: 403–408.

Johnston, C.C., Stevens, B., Craig, K.D. and Grunau, R.V.E. (1993) Developmental changes in pain expression in premature, full term, two- and four-month-old infants. *Pain*, **52**: 201–208.

Kurylyszn, N., McGrath, P.J., Cappelli, M. and Humphreys, P. (1987) Children's drawings: what they can tell us about intensity of pain? *Clinical Journal of Pain*, **2**: 155–158.

LeBaron, S. and Zeltzer, L. (1984) Assessment of acute pain and anxiety in children and adolescents by self reports, observer reports and a behaviour checklist. *Journal of Consulting and Clinical Psychology*, **52**; 729–738.

Levine, J.D. and Gordon, N.C. (1982) Pain in prelingual children and its evaluation by pain-induced vocalization. *Pain*, **14**: 85–93.

Lynn, M.R. (1986) Pain in the pediatric patient: a review of the research. *Journal of Pediatric Nursing*, **1**(3): 198–201.

Marvin, J.A. and Pomietto, M. (1991) Pain assessment in infants (0–12 months) using Neonatal Facial Action Coding System. *Journal of Pain and Symptom Management*, **6**: 193.

Mathews, J.R., McGrath, P.J. and Pigeon, H. (1993) Assessment and measurement of pain in children. In: Schechter, N.L., Berde, C.B. and Yaster, M. (eds) *Pain in Infants, Children and Adolescents*. Williams & Wilkins, Baltimore, pp. 97–111.

McCaffery, M. (1972) *Nursing Management of the Patient with Pain*. Lippincott, Philadelphia.

McCaffery, M. (1977) Pain relief for the child. *Pediatric Nursing*, July/August: 11–16.

McCaffery, M. and Beebe, A. (1989) *Pain: Clinical Manual for Nursing Practice*. Mosby, St Louis.

McGrath, P.A. (1989) Evaluating a child's pain. *Journal of Pain and Symptom Management*, **4**(4): 198–214.

McGrath, P.A. (1990) *Pain in Children: Nature, Assessment, and Treatment*. Guilford Publications, New York.

McGrath, P.J., Johnson, G., Goodman, J.T., Schillinger, J., Dunn, J. and Chapman, J. (1985) The CHEOPS: a behavioural scale to measure post operative pain in children. In: Fields, H.L., Dubner, R. and Cervero, F. (eds), *Advances in Pain Research and Therapy*. Raven Press, New York, pp. 395–402.

McGrath, P.J. and Unruh, A.M. (1987) *Pain in Children and Adolescents*. Elsevier, Amsterdam.

Melzack, R. (1975) The McGill Pain Questionnaire: major properties and scoring methods. *Pain*, **1**: 277.

Moinpour, C., Donaldson, G., Wallace, K., Hiraga, Y. and Joss, B. (1990) Parent/child agreement in rating child mouth pain. *Advances in Pain Research and Therapy*, **15**: 69–78.

Molsberry, D. (1979) *Young children's subjective quantification of pain following surgery*. Unpublished Masters thesis, University of Iowa, Iowa City.

Owens, M. (1986) Assessment of infant pain in clinical settings. *Journal of Pain and Symptom Management*, **1**(1): 29–31.

Owens, M.E. and Todt, E.H. (1984) Pain in infancy: conceptual and methodological issues. *Pain*, **20**: 77–86.

Pain Management Guidelines Panel (1992) Clinicians' quick reference guide to acute pain management in infants, children, and adolescents: operative and medical procedures. *Journal of Pain and Symptom Management*, **7**(4): 229–242.

Porter, F. (1989) Pain in the newborn. *Clinics in Perinatology*, **16**(2): 549–564.

Porter, F. (1993) Pain assessment in children: infants. In: Schechter, N.L., Berde, C.B. and Yaster, M. (eds), *Pain in Infants, Children, and Adolescents*. Williams & Wilkins, Baltimore, pp. 87–96.

Porter, F.L., Miller, R.H. and Marshall, R.E. (1986) Neonatal pain cries: effect of circumcision on acoustic features and perceived urgency. *Child Development*, **57**: 790.

Rawlings, D.J., Miller, P.A. and Engel, R.R (1980) The effect of circumcision on transcutaneous pO_2 in term infants. *American Journal of Diseases in Childhood*, **13**: 676.

Ross, D. and Ross, S. (1984) The importance of type of question, psychological climate and subject set in interviewing children about pain. *Pain*, **19**: 71–79.

Ross, D.M. and Ross, S.A. (1988) Assessment of pediatric pain. *Issues in Comprehensive Pediatric Nursing*, **11**: 73–91.

Savedra, M.C., Holzemer, W.L., Tesler, M.D. and Wilkie, D.J. (1993) Assessment of postoperation pain in children and adolescents using the Adolescent Pediatric Pain Tool. *Nursing Research*, **42**(1): 5–9.

Seers, K. (1989) Assessing pain. *Nursing Standard*, **15**(3): 33–35.

Sparshott, M. (1989) Pain and the special care baby unit. *Nursing Times*, **85**(41): 61–64.

Szyfelbein, S.K., Osgood, P.F. and Carr, D.B. (1985) The assessment of pain and plasma β-endorphin immunoactivity in burned children. *Pain*, **22**: 173.

Tarbell, S.E., Cohen, I.T. and Marsh, J.L. (1992) The Toddler–Preschooler Postoperative Pain Scale: an observational scale for measuring post-operative pain in children aged 1–5. Preliminary report. *Pain*, **50**: 273–280.

Thompson, K.L. and Varni, J.W. (1986) A developmental cognitive–biobehavioral approach to pediatric pain assessment. *Pain*, **25**; 283–296.

Tyler, D.C., Tu, A., Douhit, J. and Chapman, C.R. (1993) Toward validation of pain measurement tools for children: a pilot study. *Pain*, **52**: 301–309.

Unruh, A., McGrath, P.J., Cunningham, S.J. and Humphreys, P. (1983) Children's drawings of their pain. *Pain*, **17**: 385–392.

Van der Does, A.J. (1989) Patients' and nurses' ratings of pain and anxiety during burn wound care. *Pain*, **39**: 95–101.

Varni, J.W., Thompson, K.L. and Hanson, V. (1987) The Varni-Thompson pediatric pain questionnaire I: chronic musculoskeletal pain in juvenile rheumatoid arthritis. *Pain*, **28**: 27–38.

Wasz-Hockert, O., Lind, J., Vuorenkoski, V., Portanen, T. and Valanne, E. (1968) The infant cry: a spectrographic and auditory analysis. *Clinics in Developmental Medicine*, **29**: 9–42.

Whaley, L.F. and Wong, D.L. 61991) *Nursing Care of Infants and Children*. Mosby Year Book, St Louis.

Wilkie, D.J., Holzemer, W.L., Tesler, M.D., Ward, J.A., Paul, S.M. and Savedra, M.C. (1990) Measuring pain quality: validity and reliability of children's and adolescents' pain language. *Pain*, **41**: 151–159.

Williamson, P.S. and Williamson, R.N. (1983) Physiologic stress reduction by local anesthetic during newborn circumcision. *Pediatrics*, **71**: 36–40.

Wolff, P.H. (1974) Active language: the natural history of crying and other vocalizations in early infancy. In: Stone, L.J., Smith, H.T. and Murphy, L.B. (eds) *The Competent Infant*, Tavistock Publications, London.

Wong, D.L. and Baker, C.M. (1988) Pain in children: comparison of assessment scales. *Pediatric Nursing*, **14**: 9–17.

WHO (1980) *International Classification of Impairments, Disabilities and Handicaps*. World Health Organization, Geneva.

Zeltzer, L.K., LeBaron, S., Richie, D.M., Reed, D., Schoolfield, J. and Prohoda, T.J. (1988) Can children understand and use a rating scale to quantify symptoms? Assessment of nausea and vomiting as a model. *Journal of Consulting and Clinical Psychology*, **56**: 567–572.

Pharmacological prevention and management | 4

INTRODUCTION

Effective pain management stems from the use of a multi-method approach and it must be remembered that for the child their pain may result not only from the original disease/illness but also from the many invasive and traumatic procedures that they encounter. Pain management must attempt to ensure that pain from all sources is eliminated or reduced. Effective pain management should involve a multi-method approach. One child, for example, may find that their pain is relieved by the use of a combination of appropriate doses of opioid analgesia, relaxation techniques and massage. Alternatively another child may find benefit and derive pain control from the use of oral analgesia and distraction techniques. The situation where the nurse relies solely on the child's drug sheet for pain management is long gone and the nurse caring for the child should encourage the use of the techniques that the child and family know and trust as well as offering new approaches. Obviously nurses must be skilled and knowledgeable in all forms of pain management and should never attempt to utilize a strategy that lies outside their experience and competence. However, whilst the place of distraction, imagery, touch, massage, hypnosis and other forms of supportive or complementary care cannot, and should not, be denied, the appropriate use of pharmacological methods of pain management is of crucial importance. An essential part of the pharmacological management of the child's pain lies in delivery of skilful nursing care. Nurses involved in the administration of drugs for the relief of pain should have a sound underpinning knowledge not only of how the drugs work, what interactions should be considered, possible side-effects and contraindications but also the effects of the maturation on the disposition of the drug given.

The guiding principle in pain management stems from the belief in the child's pain and the commitment to ensure that the pain experience is diminished or controlled. It is also important to consider the nature, duration and type of pain so that appropriate analgesics can be prescribed and by an appropriate route. Since many studies have reported that children feel that injections are the 'worst hurt' steps must be taken to avoid the intramuscular route of administration.

Central to pain management is the nurse's role in the assessment and evaluation of the efficacy of any interventions and in determining the need for a change in the protocol/strategy. Nurses need to be involved in the development of pain management guidelines. Nurses also need to be willing to work within a multidisciplinary team so that a multi-dimensional approach to the challenge that pain presents can be used. The development of pain management teams such as the Paediatric Acute Pain Service described by Llewellyn (1993) provides a good example of interdisciplinary activity. Pain management should be proactive and should ensure that no child needlessly experiences pain. Pain relief, argues Jaffe (1993, p. 6), is 'poor management and relies on reacting when things are already bad'. Pre-emptive analgesia and balanced analgesia should be the principles of modern pain management (Morton, 1993). The role of pre-emptive analgesia (analgesia given prior to the noxious stimulus) is to reduce the effect of a noxious stimulus by reducing the production of pain mediators such as prostaglandins (Woolf, 1989). Balanced analgesia, on the other hand, aims to:

> block or modify the pain pathway, simultaneously, at several points . . . [to] reduce the amplification effect of a local tissue injury, producing effects on all the body's tissues via the hormonal response to injury. (Morton, 1993, p. 8).

The aim behind using pre-emptive and balanced analgesia is to provide effective analgesia, decrease morbidity, reduce the length of hospital stay and allow lower doses of analgesics to be given (Morton, 1993). Morton does not specifically discuss the psychological effects for the child but it is expected that the child and their family will be less traumatized by a regime with pain prevention rather than pain control as its central aim. Good pain management should be possible providing there is a willingness to use resources available. As Goldman and Lloyd-Thomas (1991) state:

> Our failure to adequately control pain results not from lack of suitable drugs but our own inability to use them properly. (p. 679)

Effective pharmacological management is based on assiduous attention to the four 'rights': right drug, right dose, right route and right time (Whaley and Wong, 1991).

PROFESSIONAL ATTITUDES TO PHARMACOLOGICAL MANAGEMENT

Even when health care professionals have acknowledged that the child may be experiencing pain there is an almost universal reluctance to administer appropriate analgesia, especially in respect to opioids. Beyer and Byers (1985) sum up professional fears:

At present, health care providers feel safer to undertreat than overtreat with analgesics. (p. 671)

Yaster and Desphande (1988) further state that:

Unfortunately the 'prn' order has come to mean 'give as infrequently as possible'. (p. 421)

Many myths abound which incorrectly fuel this reluctance; among these are the fear of opioid addiction (Beyers and Byers, 1985; Eland and Anderson, 1977). However, this fear is refuted by a statement made by the American Pain Society (1989):

There is no evidence that preadolescent children are at higher risk for developing psychologic dependence (addiction) than the general population when given opioids for the management of pain.

Additionally there is the issue of respiratory depression which is traditionally used as an argument for not administering opioid analgesia. This argument has been used particularly powerfully in the case of the neonate requiring pain relief. Evidence in this case strongly outweighs anecdote, with studies demonstrating that appropriate doses of opioids are safe (Beasley and Tibbalis, 1987; Dilworth and MacKellar, 1987; Webb *et al.*, 1989; Sartori *et al.*, 1990). Berde (1989) suggests that children older than 6–8 months are no more susceptible to opioid-induced respiratory depression than adults (Okkola *et al.*, 1988). Eland (1990) reports study findings in which only three of 3263 patients experienced any significant respiratory compromise. Although it may be reasonable to be concerned about the potential for respiratory depression this concern should not cloud pain management. Professionals would do well to remember that naloxone is available to reverse the effects of opioid-induced respiratory depression – not that this should make professionals complacent about the inherent dangers of using opioids.

Nurses' personal beliefs and attitudes tend to have an effect on the administration and perception of the use of 'strong analgesics'. Health care providers tend to minimize the child's pain (Davitz and Davitz, 1975). Some professionals fail to recognize and fail to respond to the importance or amount of the child's pain (Beyer and Byers, 1985; McCaffery, 1977) and many studies suggest that children are grossly under-medicated when compared to their adult counterparts (Beyer and Arandine, 1986; Mather and Mackie, 1983;

1983; Schechter *et al.*, 1986). Burokas (1985) suggests that nurses whose own children have undergone surgery are more responsive in terms of providing pain management and pain assessment.

Gadish *et al.* (1988) found that a significant number of factors affected nurses' decisions to give medication and many of these were related to the nurses' personal judgement about the pain rather than based on more objective measures.

Additionally in a study by Franck (1987) it was found that there was not a united front in terms of what constituted an indication for analgesic medication and that practices varied widely between practice settings.

> The finding that 60 of the 76 respondents believe pain medication is underused in their units indicates that nursing assessment of the need for pain medication is not being heeded. (p. 390)

Price's (1991, 1992) study of student nurses' assessment of children in pain is somewhat disturbing since the findings show that the students (not training specifically for children's nursing) tended to define pain solely in terms of the physical sensation and that half of the students used physiological signs inappropriately when assessing the child and were somewhat judgemental when describing the children's oral expressions of pain. Children were described as whinging and whining, which perhaps indicates the abyss that some nurses have to cross in order to understand what the child is experiencing. However, a study undertaken by Davis (1990) suggests that despite an improvement in the knowledge in respect to postoperative pain management nurses are not consistent in the documentation of assessment data.

PHARMACOLOGICAL APPROACHES TO PAIN MANAGEMENT

One golden rule to bear in mind with pharmacological pain management is that pain relief should not be painful, otherwise it is defeating its purpose. The type of pain will help to dictate the type of analgesia utilized. Anti-inflammatory drugs are useful in treating pain from peripheral nociceptor sensitization caused by the release of chemicals (bradykinin, substance P, prostaglandins, histamine and leukotrienes) from injured tissue. Opioids can be beneficial when the excitability of the dorsal horn neurones has been effected by afferent C fibre stimulation (Goldman and Lloyd-Thomas, 1991).

The concept of the analgesia ladder may be appropriate so that milder analgesics are used before the introduction of stronger analgesics (Alder, 1990). The analgesic ladder (or staircase as it is sometimes called) is a means of grouping analgesic drugs of a similar potency together. This aims to ensure that drugs of a similar potency are not administered if one drug from that group is already proving ineffective in pain management (Fig. 4.1). However, caution needs to be applied so that drugs with a similar potency but a

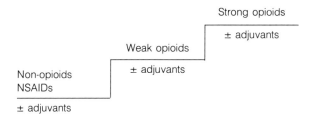

Figure 4.1 The analgesic ladder.

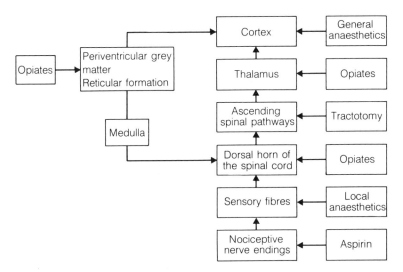

Figure 4.2 Nervous pathways mediating pain and the sites of action of analgesics. (Reproduced from Grahame-Smith and Aronson, *Oxford Textbook of Clinical Pharmacology and Drug Therapy*, pp. 458–464; by permission of Oxford University Press, 1992.)

different means of action are not ignored as a possibility before moving on and up the ladder. It should also be emphasized that the appropriate rung of the ladder is chosen in order to prevent and/or relieve a child's pain. Indeed it is also important to ensure that combinations of drugs from different rungs can often be used together very effectively. Additionally these agents can be used in conjunction with other techniques. If this view is taken the ladder perhaps gets rather confusing.

ANALGESICS

Specific groups of analgesic act on specific sites within the nervous system. Understanding the target site for their actions provides a rationale for their administration so that the most appropriate drug or combination of drugs can be used. Analgesics can target:

- nociceptive nerve endings;
- nerves which are stimulated by mediators of pain;
- the sensory nerves which are responsible for transfer of impulses to the spinal cord;
- the dorsal horn of the spinal cord responsible for receiving the impulse from the sensory nerves, processing the signal and passing it on via the ascending nerve pathways in the spinal cord;
- the thalamus where processing occurs; and
- the cortex where the sensation is experienced.

Signals can then descend to the dorsal horn of the spinal cord either to inhibit or to facilitate activity (Fig. 4.2).

There are basically two main categories of analgesics: the opioids and the non-opioids. These categories can be further broken down.

Opioids $\begin{cases} \text{non-synthetic or semi-synthetic compounds related to morphine} \\ \text{synthetic compounds not related to morphine} \end{cases}$

Non-opioids $\begin{cases} \text{aspirin and related salicylates} \\ \text{paracetamol} \end{cases}$

The opioids act as either complete or partial agonists at opioid receptors in the brain, spinal cord and periphery. The non-opioids are generally thought to act peripherally although they may have some central effects (McQuay, 1992).

OPIOIDS

Opioids are drugs with a morphine-like effect. Opioids are classified in terms of their receptor-binding properties as agonists, antagonists and mixed agonist–antagonists. Opioids bind to multiple opioid receptor sites at the ends of the nerves in the central nervous system (CNS), and at spinal and supraspinal levels. Four primary opioid receptor types found in the CNS are of real importance in the clinical use of opioids. The mu (μ) receptor site is located in specific areas of the brain, including the thalamus and in the substantia gelatinosa of the spinal cord. It is concerned with activity related to spinal and supraspinal analgesia, respiratory depression, decrease in gastrointestinal motility, euphoria and physical dependence. The kappa (κ) receptor sites are located in specific areas of the brain such as the hypothalamus. The sites have effects on spinal analgesia, sedation and inhibition of release of antidiuretic hormone. The delta (δ) sites are located in the brain, including the deep cortex and the amygdala. This site has effects on analgesia and euphoria. The sigma (σ) receptor site has effects on hallucinations and psychomotor stimulation.

Opioids given to relieve pain bind to the opioid receptor site, where the action may be agonist (pure or partial) or antagonist. Agonists bind to the opioid receptor sites and they 'switch' the activity on (the activity being analgesia). Pure agonists bind tightly with the receptor sites and the result is a high level of activity at the receptor site. The partial agonists produce a reduced level of activity as they do not bind so tightly to the receptor sites.

Antagonists have an opposite effect since when they bind to specific receptor sites they effectively block the activity or they displace the agonist at the receptor site and stop the activity. This is important in cases where the opioid is causing respiratory depression and there is a clinical need to stop the activity of morphine, for example. The administration of a pure antagonist such as naloxone will reverse the respiratory depression and the analgesia. Naloxone antagonizes the μ, κ and σ sites. The opioid agonist–antagonists occupy the κ site and result in pain relief, with fewer problems with respiratory depression (McCaffery and Beebe, 1989) (Table 4.1).

Table 4.1 Action of opioids at receptor subtypes

Agent	Mu (μ)	Kappa (κ)	Sigma (σ)
Morphine Fentanyl Codeine	Agonist	Agonist	Minimal effects
Naloxone	Antagonist	Antagonist	Antagonist

Morphine

Morphine is the gold standard for analgesia against which all other analgesics are measured. Morphine can be administered orally, intramuscularly, intravenously, intrathecally, epidurally, rectally and subcutaneously. Perhaps the biggest not fully acknowledged problem with morphine usage is not related to the much-discussed side-effects but that inappropriately small doses are prescribed at intervals which are too long for children's individual needs. Yaster and Deshpande (1988) cite Mather and Phillips (1986), who propose:

> Rational use of opioids requires a flexible, patient oriented approach to allow for variability in individual pain experience and tolerance, as well as a knowledge of both the beneficial and adverse effects of the particular drug being used. (p. 423)

However, respiratory depression is a legitimate concern with morphine as it reduces the sensitivity of brain stem respiratory centres to arterial carbon dioxide content ($paCO_2$). Yaster and Deshpande (1988) state that infants of less than 1–2 months of age are particularly vulnerable in this respect.

Infants with their incomplete blood–brain barriers may experience a more profound effect from the administration of morphine than older children, and infants of less than 1 month have been shown to have a prolonged elimination half-life when compared with older children and adults. Neonates also have a reduced plasma binding capacity and therefore require only small doses (Koren *et al.*, 1985). However, Yaster and Maxwell (1993) provide a useful comment when they state:

> the hesitancy in prescribing and administering morphine to children less that one year may not be warranted. On the other hand, *the use of any opioid in children less than 2 months old must be limited to a monitored setting.* (p. 155)

Table 4.2 Physiological effects of opioids by organ system (Yaster and Maxwell, 1993)

I. Central nervous system
    A. Analgesia
    B. Sedation
    C. Dysphoria and euphoria
    D. Nausea and vomiting
    E. Miosis
    F. Seizures
    G. Psychotomimetic behaviours, excitation
II. Respiratory system
    A. Antitussive
    B. Respiratory depression (decreased minute ventilation)
       1. Decreased respiratory rate
       2. Decreased tidal volume
       3. Decreased ventilatory response to carbon dioxide
    C. Bronchospasm
       1. Morphine releases histamine
III. Cardiovascular system
    A. Heart rate
       1. Bradycardia (fentanyl, morphine)
       2. Tachycardia (meperidine)
    B. Minimal effects on cardiac output
    C. Vasodilation, venodilation
       1. Morphine > > > other opioids, ?histamine effect
IV. Gastrointestinal system
    A. Decreased intestinal motility and peristalsis
       1. Therapy for diarrhoea
       2. Side-effect = constipation
    B. Increased sphincter tone
       1. Sphincter of Oddi
       2. Ileocolic
V. Urinary system
    A. Increased tone
       1. Ureters
       2. Bladder
       3. Detrusor muscles of the bladder

Morphine, along with the other opioids, produces a number of side-effects on the systems of the body. The nurse should be aware of all of these so that assessment for side-effects is made knowledgeably and effectively (Table 4.2).

The clinical signs of incipient respiratory depression associated with morphine that the nurse must be alert for include drowsiness, small tidal volumes and small pupils.

Nurses should make frequent assessments not only of the effectiveness of the beneficial analgesic effects of the morphine but should also ensure that the child's vital signs are monitored, with particular care being taken in assessing and documenting the child's respiratory rate and rhythm and an assessment of the child's sedation level. The use of an oxygen saturation monitor can be helpful in providing an early indication of respiratory depression and apnoea monitors should be considered for children under 6 months of age.

Since every child's pain is individual and their response to analgesia is individual, morphine dosage (as with any other analgesic) should be carefully titrated against analgesic effects and potential side-effects, especially when the intravenous route is used. When given intravenously it passes the blood–brain barrier within 6–10 minutes, which means that the peak activity time and thus the peak time for possible side-effects occurs about 10 minutes after administration. The nurse must assess the child very carefully in the first 10 minutes after a bolus dose of intravenous morphine. After this period of time titration of the dose can occur. Morton (1993) proposes dosage regimes which can act as a guide (Table 4.3). However, any such guide should not be

Table 4.3 Opioid techniques (Morton, 1993)

Intravenous morphine
Concentration 1 mg/kg in 50 ml
Bolus dose 0.1–0.2 mg/kg
Infusion rate, age   0–1 month: 5 µg/kg per hour
                     1<3 months: 10 µg/kg per hour
                     >3 months: 20 µg/kg per hour

Subcutaneous morphine
Concentration 1 mg/kg in 20 ml
Bolus dose 0.1–0.2 mg/kg
Infusion rate, age   0–1 month: 5 µg/kg per hour
                     1<3 months: 10 µg/kg per hour
                     >3 months: 20 µg/kg per hour

Patient-controlled analgesia
Concentration 1 mg/kg in 50 ml
Bolus dose 20 µg/kg
Lockout interval 5 min
Background infusion nil

used too prescriptively and a degree of flexibility is vital, especially in relation to patient-controlled analgesia. Subcutaneous morphine can be used in the management of severe pain associated with terminal malignancy (Williams, 1987) and in postoperative pain (Lavies and Wandless, 1989). Subcutaneous morphine eliminates the need for either intramuscular injection or intravenous access and it is managed more readily at home for children needing long-term pain care (Miser *et al.*, 1983).

Fentanyl

Fentanyl is a useful, synthetically derived opiate which is given intravenously and has both a rapid onset (190–120 seconds) and a short duration (up to 40 minutes), which makes it a useful analgesic agent for the management of procedural pain such as bone marrow aspiration, wound drainage and manipulation of fractures (Waters, 1992; Roop Moyer and Howe, 1991).

Fentanyl (2–4 μg/kg per hour) given via infusion has been used in neonates receiving mechanical ventilation and is said to be effective with those neonates at risk from pulmonary hypertension (Goldman and Lloyd-Thomas, 1991). Fentanyl is approximately 80 times as potent as morphine (Roop Moyer and Howe, 1991). The side-effects of fentanyl are similar to morphine but tend to occur only with large doses and too rapid administration. However, chest wall rigidity has been reported with too rapid an infusion which may make ventilation problematic or impossible (Berde *et al.*, 1990a, Yaster and Deshpande, 1988). Should this occur a muscle relaxant such as pancuronium needs to be administered to treat the rigidity.

Fentanyl can also be given by the oral transmucosal route as a 'fentanyl lollipop' which has proved popular with children who have used it, although side-effects such as facial pruritus, nausea and vomiting have been reported (Gaukroger, 1993a). Schechter *et al.* (1990) report the use of fentanyl lollipops with nine children (aged 3–18 years) who underwent bone marrow aspirator lumbar puncture. The study showed that the older children gained better pain relief than the younger children but that no child experienced changes to respiratory rate, oxygen saturation or blood pressure. Vomiting was a side-effect with three children. The authors suggest that fentanyl lollipop could be a 'more humane approach' to utilize compared with other approaches.

NON-STEROIDAL ANTI-INFLAMMATORY DRUGS

These drugs have analgesic, anti-inflammatory and antipyretic properties. Although their total mode of action is as yet unclear, the inhibition of prostaglandin synthesis (Grahame-Smith and Aronson, 1992) and in some cases antagonizing the effects of prostaglandins at receptor sites (McGrath and Unruh, 1987) are implicated. They reduce the metabolism of arachidonic acid to prostaglandins. Arachidonic acid, which is normally stored within cell membranes, is released when the membranes are disrupted, such as occurs in local injury and inflammation. Prostaglandins are responsible for sensitizing nerve endings to pain but do not cause pain in their own right.

Acetylsalicylic acid (aspirin)

Aspirin is a well-established drug that should not be used for children under the age of 12 years old owing to the increased risk/association with Reye's syndrome. Reye's syndrome is a rare syndrome that appears to be associated with the use of aspirin. It is a potentially fatal disease that primarily attacks the brain and the liver. Additionally aspirin inhibits platelet aggregation and care should be taken therefore in the administration of this commonly available drug.

Diclofenac and keterolac

These agents are reported to have fewer side-effects than aspirin (Maunuksela, 1993). Morton (1993) proposes that these drugs 'hold great promise as pre-emptive analgesics for incorporating in balanced analgesic regimes' (p. 9).

Aspirin and the other non-steroidal anti-inflammatory drugs (NSAIDS) have traditionally been the first line of pharmacological management for children with juvenile rheumatoid arthritis. Page (1991) reports that a regime of NSAIDS is the 'only one necessary for 60–75% of cases'. However, there is no firm evidence as yet to prove their efficacy in the management of acute pain. Care should be taken with these drugs as some children may react to diclofenac and keterolac.

ACETAMINOPHEN (PARACETAMOL)

Paracetamol has no anti-inflammatory properties but it has analgesic and antipyretic properties. It is thought that this effect is achieved through selective inhibition of prostaglandin synthesis in some tissue. Paracetomol is now the most frequently used analgesic for mild to moderate pain for children. It is safe if used within the therapeutic range. It is readily available in appropriate child formulations and is generally well accepted by children.

EMLA CREAM (5%) (EUTECTIC MIXTURE OF LOCAL ANAESTHETICS)

EMLA cream is now a popular and effective means of reducing the pain associated with venepuncture or venous cannulation. It is a 1 : 1 oil–water emulsion of a eutectic mixture of lidocaine and prilocaine. The mixture anaesthetizes the skin very readily and once applied under an occlusive dressing it takes a minimum of 60 minutes to be effective, although 90 minutes is often recommended (Wahstedt *et al.*, 1984). Morton (1993) reports the effectiveness of EMLA cream with other procedures such as lumbar puncture, division of prepucial adhesions, skin grafts and in the preparation of the skin prior to infiltration of local anaesthetic around small surface lesions that require excision.

Although very effective in diminishing the physical pain of many procedures it does require to be administered at least 60 minutes before the procedure and this is an area in which the nurse can ensure that preplanning can result in application well in advance. Children do not generally appear to become upset with the application of the cream and again careful preparation of the child and telling them why they are having the cream applied is a helpful part of the psychological preparation of the child for any procedure. For children awaiting venepuncture and/or venous cannulation more than one site should be prepared in case problems are experienced with the first site, so that another prepared area is available for use. Care needs to be taken in using EMLA with neonates since prilocaine can be absorbed in the newborn and can result in methaemoglobinaemia. Neonates are reported to be particularly susceptible to low levels of the enzyme methaemoglobin reductase (Goldman and Lloyd-Thomas, 1991).

Lidocaine gel and ointment can be used to minimize pain associated with urethral catheterization and circumcision and the spray can be used in endotracheal intubation.

PATIENT-CONTROLLED ANALGESIA

Patient-controlled analgesia (PCA) is an increasingly popular method of ensuring that the child has a pain-free recovery. Although originally used in the management of postoperative pain, PCA is now used for many different types of acute and chronic pain (Bender *et al.*, 1990; Roop Moyer and Howe, 1991; Schechter *et al.*, 1988). Opioids are commonly administered by this method. PCA was developed during the 1970s in an attempt to allow patients to control their own analgesic requirements and thus maintain pain relief. PCA allows the child to self-administer small, frequent, intravenous boluses of analgesia via a specially designed pump. The child can operate a pump by a hand-held trigger that signals the pump to deliver a preset amount of the drug via their infusion line, provided that the lock-out period has elapsed. The lock-out period or interval prevents potential overdose as it will not allow the child actively to trigger the machine for a set period of time after they last used the trigger. The lock-out period is specially programmed into the machine.

Most PCA devices allow four different approaches to analgesic management: continuous infusion, interval doses only, continuous infusion with interval doses, and continuous infusion with interval doses and bolus doses (Bender *et al.*, 1990). However, some confusion may result from the seemingly complex terminology and the nurse must ensure that they completely understand what is meant by individual terms within their own practice.

The basal rate or background infusion is the amount of drug that is continuously infused as a background analgesia regardless of the child's 'additional' demands. The interval dose is the amount of drug that has been pre-programmed into the PCA device that the child can deliver themselves. The lock-out interval is the preset time during which the child cannot receive another dose. Bolus doses may additionally be prescribed so that the nurse can deliver a prescribed dose if the child is not receiving adequate pain control. However, the need for bolus doses should indicate that the background infusion and/or the interval dose and/or lock-out time need reassessing.

Apart from giving the child 'control' over their analgesia, which is important psychologically in its own right, PCA eliminates the peaks and troughs that are recognized to occur with more routine approaches to pain relief, such as in the use of intramuscular injections or via the oral route (Bender *et al.*, 1990). The decision either to administer or not to administer the analgesic via a PCA system may be one of the choices that the child can take or help to take in respect of their pain management and analgesia. The issue of control is important since it will be the child who, within safe, preset parameters, decides when they require analgesia and then administers it rather than having to report their pain to the doctor or the nurse, who then may or may not decide that they 'deserve' analgesia and then has to go away from the child to get the drug before administering it. The decision is the child's and one that they are usually glad to take responsibility for. On occasions, if the child is too young to understand the concept of PCA the parents may be the people most appropriate to control the analgesia. This, however, remains an area that is somewhat controversial and requires both further study and careful consideration of parameters that need to be set for the very young child. Alternatively a nurse-controlled analgesic system has been used in a similar manner. PCA was initially developed for use by adults and then was trialled with adolescents and has been used with children as young as 4 years of age (Gaukroger, 1993b). Gillespie and Morton (1992) report the successful use of PCA in children as young as 5 years. Dodd *et al.* (1988) report that PCA has been used successfully within a study of eight paediatric patients aged 6–16 years using morphine. Rodgers *et al.* (1988) also report successful use of PCA in children undergoing either thoracotomy or major abdominal surgery. Gaukroger (1993b) reports that in a study of 1000 children PCA was used well by the majority, although some of the 4-year-olds needed additional support and/or teaching. The 5–6-year-olds mostly were able to use PCA unaided and the children older than 7 years were almost all able to use PCA.

Berde *et al.* (1991) report the generally successful use of PCA in children (aged 7–19 years) after elective orthopaedic surgery. Other studies report generally successful use of PCA in children over the age of 7 years in a variety of postoperative situations (Rauen and Ho, 1989; Bender *et al.*, 1990; Webb *et al.*, 1989).

One crucial aspect of nursing management in respect to PCA is that of initial assessment to determine if the child is suitable for PCA. A number of criteria should be considered prior to introducing the child to the possible use of PCA. The child should be old enough to understand that by pushing the button when they feel pain the machine will generally give them some medicine to take their pain away. Explanations of this should be age appropriate and the concept of the lock-out also needs explaining clearly so that the child understands this aspect. The child and their family should be reassured that the machine will not replace the nurse but provides a safe and effective means of managing pain that frees some nursing time so that other pain management strategies and care can be given. Bender *et al.* (1990) cite a study by Levi and Osborne (1986) which suggests that as much as 25% time was saved through the use of PCA compared with other forms of analgesic administration. Panfilli *et al.* (1988) report that the time saved by the use of PCA allows greater opportunity for the use of non-pharmaceutical approaches to support and care for the child.

The child should be told of any time lag that they are likely to experience in the relief of their pain after they have pushed the button. Children should be encouraged to tell the nurses about how effective (or indeed ineffective) the PCA is and to report any difficulties or concerns that they have. They should also be able to manipulate the trigger button – some machines have quite large hand-held devices, originally designed and suited to adult hands, that prove problematic for little fingers and hands.

Good explanations about the degree of pain relief is important initially as the child needs to be told that although they should not experience any unpleasant pain they may experience some discomfort (Gaukroger, 1993b). These episodes of discomfort are times in which the other supportive measures such as distraction, imagery and massage can be of real help. Roop Moyer and Howe (1991) discuss that from their clinical experience some children may be frightened of the potential for overdosage of the drug and of becoming addicted. This phenomenon has also been reported by Gaukroger (1993b) and Bender *et al.* (1990). The principles of assessment for the use of PCA need to be considered carefully and a checklist of some type needs to be 'ticked off' to ensure that the PCA is right for the child and the child is right for PCA (Table 4.4).

The advantages of PCA are extensive for the child and children who have used PCA have generally reported a high level of satisfaction with it. Webb *et al.* (1989) in a study of 15 11–18-year-olds (a further 15 were in the control group) found that 73% would want to use PCA again and eight of the

Table 4.4 Principles of assessment for use of PCA

Child has an understanding of cause and effect

Child can handle the PCA trigger button/device

Child wants to use PCA

Child can understand that pushing the button will not necessarily always give them their medicine

Child understands the pain assessment tool

Child understands that the nurse is still there to help them, especially if the PCA 'doesn't work'

Child should understand that the PCA should help their pain but it should not make them very, very sleepy (sedated) (although they can obviously go to sleep)

Child can explain to the nurse about how PCA works to show they have grasped the essentials

---

children compared it favourably with other methods of analgesia administration. Parents have also found that PCA was a satisfactory method. The best advantage reported by the children to PCA was that they did not have to wait.

In a report of practice by Bender *et al.* (1990) of the use of PCA in the management of the postoperative period after spinal fusion children found it preferable to intramuscular injections and this is also reported by Berde *et al.* (1991). The major advantage is the elimination of the fear associated with intramuscular injections. In Webb *et al.*'s (1989) study the pattern of drug requirements is similar to that seen in adult patients: an initial 'heavy' demand for analgesia in the immediate postoperative period with a steady decrease in the subsequent days, the children in the PCA group needing less analgesia than those in the control group from day 3 onwards. This tailing off of morphine requirements is seen in Rauen and Ho's (1989) study of 20 female children (10–19 years) who used PCA after spinal surgery. Success of PCA depends on the preparation of the child and the correct prescription of the drug and programming of the PCA device. Lock-out intervals of between 5 and 15 minutes are advocated (Gaukroger, 1993a; Bender *et al.*, 1990; Goldman and Lloyd-Thomas, 1991).

It is vital that the nurse is fully involved in caring for the child with PCA. Assessment, not only of pain management but also of how successfully the child is managing the 'technology' and if they seem to be confident with it, is vital. The nurse must also observe the child for signs of potential opioid overload, including assessing respiratory rate, pulse, consciousness level/level of sedation, nausea and vomiting and the volume of drug administered. These parameters allow the nurse to judge, along with the child's own reports of pain through the use of an appropriate pain assessment tool, the success or otherwise of the intervention. Should any side-effects occur the PCA will need to be adjusted or even discontinued (temporarily or completely). If the child's PCA needs to be discontinued then careful explanations of why this is so need to be given to the child, who ultimately has lost control of something very precious – their ability to control their pain.

Although well accepted by children PCA does still produce reports of side-effects. Reports of respiratory depression are infrequent. Respiratory depression was not seen to be a major problem by Rauen and Ho (1989), Berde *et al.* (1991) or Gaukroger (1993a), Webb *et al.* (1989) and most authors report it as being a very safe means of administering opioids. However, Berde *et al.* (1991) and Gaukroger (1993a) discuss the level of sedation as sometimes being either too little or too much. Rauen and Ho (1989) reported in their study two children who exhibited somewhat confused or disoriented behaviour; one of the children had hallucinations which subsided within 12 hours – she was commenced on oral analgesia after the PCA had been stopped.

Some studies measured the ratio of the number of successful injections against attempts at injection. Rauen and Ho (1989) reported that the range of successful attempts was 33–95%. This is obviously an issue that needs further consideration, questions need to be asked about why the number of apparently unsuccessful attempts can be so high and to see if this can be decreased by improved preparation or whether or not the infusion is set appropriately for that individual child's needs. As with any system a number of potential hazards exist and although the systems are designed to be fail-safe they are not completely idiot- or child-proof (Table 4.5).

Overall PCA is reported to be a safe and effective method of pain management, provided all the staff involved have an adequate level of knowledge and skill with the technique and that time is spent teaching their child and their family about the use of PCA, preferably well before the system is used (Berde *et al.*, 1991). The nursing time that is 'saved' by the use of PCA can be reinvested in the use of other nursing measures to help support the child and family.

Table 4.5 Potential hazards associated with PCA (developed from Waters, 1992; Webb *et al.*, 1989; Gaukroger, 1993a)

Improper loading of the pump
Improper drawing up of syringe contents
Improper programming of the pump
Syringes cracking/breaking on insertion
PCA trigger button falling on the floor and administering inadvertent dose
Overdosage if background infusion inappropriately high
Drug accumulating in the intravenous tubing if there is no one-way valve in the line or if it is incorrectly placed
'Bolus' dose given if the line is flushed through with another fluid
Equipment malfunction

REGIONAL ANAESTHESIA

Anaesthetics used in regional anaesthesia work by blocking sodium channels in the axonal membrane, which inhibits sodium conductance. This results in a reduction in the rate and degree of depolarization of the nerve cell and thus prevents the propagation of the action potential. They basically produce a 'transient, reversible blockade of nerve function' (McQuay, 1992). Children and their parents must be prepared appropriately if local anaesthetics are to be used as the child may become distressed by the motor block and the lack of sensation. Regional anaesthesia for the management of pain is becoming an increasingly popular approach as it produces effective analgesia for a range of pain situations (Yaster and Maxwell, 1989). Local anaesthesia has been used to good effect in the management of procedural pain and it is an effective strategy for use within the day care surgery situation and for the management of major surgery (Lloyd-Thomas, 1990). It is of value with a wide age range and Yaster (1987) is categorical in his belief in local anaesthesia in regards to the use of lidocaine in the care of neonates:

Local infiltration of the skin is so safe that there is little, if any, reason ever to perform a cutdown for vascular access without its use. (p. 395)

However, it should be noted that children have a different pharmokinetic response to local anaesthesia than adults and tend to absorb and eliminate regional anaesthetic drugs faster than adults, although they may display a prolonged terminal elimination half-life (Lloyd-Thomas, 1990).

Although regional anaesthesia has been used for 30 years in children it has received closer attention over the past 10 years as it provides a good alternative to other methods of pain management (Ecoffey, 1990; Desparmet *et al.*, 1990; Lloyd-Thomas, 1990; Desparmet, 1993). Regional anaesthesia and analgesia provide a safe and effective alternative to the utilization of other techniques (Dalens, 1993). Sethna and Wilder (1993) report that regional anaesthesia can be used for pain control, prophylactic pain management, diagnostic purposes and for prognostic effects. Ecoffey (1990) reports a wide range of beneficial effects (Table 4.6) during the intraoperative and postoperative period.

Table 4.6 Beneficial effects of regional blocks (developed from Ecoffey, 1990)

Allows suppression of undesired reflexes such as laryngospasm

Can provide prolonged postoperative pain relief using anaesthetic, analgesic agents or a combination of both which can be 'topped up'

Decreased narcotic and non-narcotic requirements

Decreased use of muscle relaxants

Faster recovery to the child's normal state of alertness and enhanced recovery and healing

Improved mobility postoperatively

Child is calmer due to the effectiveness of the technique

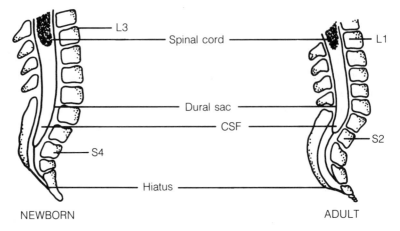

Figure 4.3 Anatomical differences between the spine of children and adults.

Regional anaesthesia offers improved pain management for both children and neonates (Lloyd-Thomas, 1990). Children and infants present unique physiological and anatomical considerations when compared with adults (Fig. 4.3). Anatomically the tip of the spinal cord is at L3 with the dura at S3 at birth, and at L1–2 by the age of 12 months with the dura at S2. This needs to be taken into account when inserting the needle or catheter. The infant's sacrum is flat and the bony landmarks are usually readily seen and located. Additionally the extradural fat is gelatinous, loosely packed and is characterized by spaces, whereas adults have tightly packed fat divided by fibrous strands; this structure allows a greater longitudinal spread of the solutions injected into the space. Children under the age of 6 years demonstrate marked cardiovascular stability (Lloyd-Thomas, 1990), whereas adults and older children can demonstrate significant clinical hypotension after epidural or spinal anaesthesia (Ecoffey, 1990). Regional anaesthesia can be divided into two main categories: central and peripheral (Table 4.7). Regional anaesthesia and analgesia are reported as being successful not only during the intra- and postoperative period but also in the management of reflex sympathetic dystrophy, myofascial pain syndromes, cancer pain, cystic fibrosis pain and sickle cell crisis pain (Sethna and Wilder, 1993).

The **caudal route** is widely used as it is simple, safe and effective as a means of providing analgesia, although some studies would suggest that it is not suitable for re-injection due to proximity of the insertion site to the anus, which increases the risk of infection (Ecoffey, 1990). However, providing the time is limited to three days, Desparmet (1993) reports that the site can be used to deliver prolonged pain relief. It is suitable for use with all ages, including neonates (Lloyd-Thomas, 1990). It can be used in conjunction with general anaesthesia for analgesia during the intra- and

Table 4.7 Types of regional anaesthesia

Central blocks
 Caudal
 Epidural
 Spinal

Peripheral
Upper extremity
 Brachial plexus
 Axillary
Lower extremity
 Penile
 Ilioinguinal
 Iliohypogastric
 Intercostal
Wound infiltration

postoperative period for surgery and procedures involving the lower limbs, abdominal surgery below the level of the umbilicus as well as genitourinary and the anoperineum. Opioids can be used via the caudal route although great care must be taken in monitoring the child owing to the risk of respiratory depression (Desparmet, 1993).

Epidural blocks are now possible with a wide age range of children owing to the availability of paediatric-sized epidural catheters, which are small enough to allow even infants to be safely managed (Ecoffey, 1990; Desparmet, 1993). This route is reported as being successful in managing postoperative pain with bupivicaine infusion (Desparmet *et al.*, 1987; Ecoffey, 1990) and with opioids such as morphine (Desparmet *et al.*, 1990. Ecoffey, 1990) with opioids and local anaesthetics (Desparmet, 1990) and fentanyl and bupivicaine (Berde *et al.*, 1990a). Possible side-effects when using opioids include urinary retention, nausea, pruritus and a potential risk of delayed respiratory depression. The nurse must carefully observe for these potential problems.

Spinal blocks are not widely used in children owing to a reported high incidence of headache (Desparmet, 1993). However, it is a good approach to use in the management of high-risk infants such as premature and ex-premature infants who are especially prone to apnoea (Mahé and Ecoffey, 1988; Lloyd-Thomas, 1990; Ecoffey, 1993).

Peripheral nerve blocks are of value in the management of analgesia during the intra- and postoperative period and provide a localized area of anaesthesia. Dalens (1993) reports that regional blockade is 'better than any other mode of therapy' in respect to this situation. Most peripheral blocks are established whilst the child is anaesthetized so as not to unnecessarily frighten them with a procedure involving a needle (Lloyd-Thomas,1990; Dalens, 1993). The use of an electric nerve stimulator can ensure correct placement of the needle for the nerve block. As with central blocks the child needs good psychological preparation by the nurse so that they are not frightened by the persistent motor and sensory blockade. However, Dalens (1993) reports that dilute concentrations of local anaesthetics can achieve a sensory blockade without having too major an impact on motor function/blockade. A variety of blocks can be used (see Table 4.7) and infiltration of the wound itself has proved successful. Williamson and Williamson (1983) also found firm evidence of the effectiveness of using lidocaine as a local anaesthetic and suggest its use could be widened to allow procedures such as insertion of chest drains. Peripheral blockade is an important technique in the management and care of the child in pain, and importantly, it is of value in pain prevention.

REFERENCES

Alder, S. (1990) Taking children at their word: pain control in paediatrics. *Professional Nurse*, May: 398–402.

American Pain Society (1989) *Principles of analgesic use in the treatment of acute pain or chronic cancer pain.* American Pain Society, Washington.

Beasley, S.W. and Tibbalis, J. (1987) Efficacy and safety of continuous morphine infusion for postoperative analgesic in the paediatric surgical ward. *Australian and New Zealand Journal of Surgery*, **57**: 233–237.

Bender, L.H., Weaver, K. and Edwards, W. (1990) Postoperative patient-controlled analgesia in children. *Pediatric Nursing*, **16**(6): 549–554.

Berde, C. (1989) Regional analgesia in the management of chronic pain in children. *Journal of Pain and Symptom Management*, **4**(4): 232–237.

Berde, C., Albin, A. and Glazer, J. (1990a) Report of the subcommittee of disease related pain in childhood cancer. *Pediatrics*, **86**(65): 818–825.

Berde, C.B., Sethna, N.F., Yemen, T.A. *et al.* (1990b) Continuous epidural bupivicaine–fentanyl infusion in children following ureteral reimplantation (Abstract). *Anesthesia and Analgesia*, **73**: A1128.

Berde, C.B., Lehn, B.M., Yee, J.D., Sethna, N.F. and Russo, D. (1991) Patient-controlled analgesia in children and adolescents: a randomized, prospective comparison with intramuscular morphine for postoperative analgesia. *Journal of Pediatrics*,**118**: 460–466.

Beyer, J. and Arandine, C. (1986) Content validity of an instrument to measure young children's perception of the intensity of their pain. *Journal of Pediatric Nursing*, **1**(6): 386–395.

Beyer, J.E. and Byers, M.L. (1985) Knowledge of pediatric pain: the state of the art. *Children's Health Care*, **13**(4): 150–159.

Burokas, L. (1985) Factors affecting nurses' decisions to medicate patients after surgery. *Heart and Lung*, **14**(4): 373–379.

Dalens, B. (1993) Peripheral nerve blockade in the management of postoperative pain in children. In: Schechter, N.L., Berde, C.B. and Yaster, M. (eds), *Pain in Infants, Children, and Adolescents*. Williams & Wilkins, Baltimore, pp. 261–280.

Davis, K.L. (1990) Postoperative pain in toddlers: nurses' assessment and intervention. In: Tyler, D.C.and Krane, E.J. (eds), *Advances in Pain Research Therapy*, Vol. 15. Raven Press, New York, pp. 53–61.

Davitz, L. and Davitz, J. (1975) How nurses view patient suffering. *Registered Nurse*, **38**: 69–74.

Desparmet, J.F. (1993) Central blocks in children and adolescents. In: Schechter, N.L., Berde, C.B. and Yaster, M. (eds), *Pain in Infants, Children, and Adolescents*. Williams & Wilkins, Baltimore, pp. 245–260.

Desparmet, J., Desmazs, N., Mazoit, X. and Ecoffey, C. (1990) Evolution of regional anesthesia in a pediatric surgical practice. In: Tyler, D.C. and Krane, E.J. (eds), *Advances in Pain Research Therapy*, Vol. 15, Raven Press, New York, pp. 201–207.

Desparmet, J., Meiselman, C., Barre, J. and Saint-Maurice, C. (1987) Continuous epidural infusion of bupivicaine for post-operative pain relief in children. *Anesthesiology*, **67**: 108–110.

Dilworth, N.M. and MacKellar, A. (1987) Pain relief for the pediatric surgical patient. *Journal of Pediatric Surgery*, **22**: 264–266.

Dodd, E., Wang, J.M. and Rauck, R.L. (1988) Patient controlled analgesia for post-surgical pediatric patients ages 6–16 years. *Anesthesiology*, **69**: A372.

Ecoffey, C. (1990) Regional anesthesia techniques in children. In: Tyler, D.C. and Krane, E.J. (eds), *Advances in Pain Research Therapy*, Vol. 15. Raven Press, New York, pp. 157–165.

Eland, J.M. (1990) Pain in children. *Nursing Clinics of North America*, **25**(4): 871–874.

Eland, J.M. and Anderson, J.E. (1977) The experience of pain in children. In: Jacox, A.K. (ed.), *Pain: A Sourcebook for Nurses and Other Health Professionals*. Little, Brown & Co., Boston, pp.453–471.

Franck, L.S. (1987) A national survey of the assessment and treatment of pain and agitation in the neonatal intensive care unit. *Journal of Obstetrics, Gynecology and Neonatal Nursing*, **16**(6): 387–393.

Gadish, H.S., Gonzalez, J.L. and Hayes, J.S. (1988) Factors affecting nurses' decisions to administer pediatric pain medication postoperatively. *Journal of Pediatric Nursing: Nursing Care of Children and Families*, 3(6): 383–390.

Gaukroger, P.B. (1993a) Novel techniques of analgesic delivery. In: Schechter, N.L., Berde, C.B. and Yaster, M. (eds), *Pain in Infants, Children, and Adolescents*. Williams & Wilkins, Baltimore, pp. 195–201.

Gaukroger, P.B. (1993b) Patient-controlled analgesia in children. In: Schechter, N.L., Berde, C.B. and Yaster, M. (eds), *Pain in Infants, Children, and Adolescents*. Williams & Wilkins, Baltimore, pp. 203–211.

Gillespie, J. and Morton, N. (1992) Patient-controlled analgesia for children: a review. *Pediatric Anaesthesia*, **2**: 51–59.

Goldman, A. and Lloyd-Thomas, A.R. (1991) Pain management in children. In: Wells, J.C.D. and Woolf, C.J. (eds), *Pain Mechanisms and Management*, Churchill Livingstone, Edinburgh, pp. 676–689.

Grahame-Smith, D.G. and Aronson, J.K. (1992) *Oxford Textbook of Clinical Pharmacology and Drug Therapy*. Oxford University Press, Oxford.

Jaffe, P. (1993) Relief only when desperate. *Nursing Standard Supplement*, **7**(25): 6.

Koren, G., Butt, W., Chinyanga, H., Soldin, S., Tan, Y.-K., and Pape, K. (1985) Postoperative morphine infusion in newborn infants: assessment of disposition characteristics and safety. *Journal of Pediatrics*, **107**(6): 963–967.

Lavies, N.G. and Wandless, J.G. (1989) Subcutaneous morphine in children: taking the sting out of postoperative analgesia. *Anaesthesia*, **44**: 1000–1001.

Levi, P. and Osborne, J. (1986) Patient controlled analgesia: traditional versus mechanical. *Journal of Nursing Administration*, **16**(9): 18–19.

Llewellyn, N. (1993) A.P.S. A multidisciplinary team. *Nursing Standard Supplement*, **7**(25): 7.

Lloyd-Thomas, A.R. (1990) Pain management in paediatric patients. *British Journal of Anaesthesia*, **64**: 85–104.

Mahé, V. and Ecoffey, C. (1988) Spinal anaesthesia with isobaric bupivicaine in infants. *Anesthesiology*, **68**: 601–603.

Mather, L.E. and Mackie, J. (1983) The incidence of postoperative pain in children. *Pain*, **15**: 271–282.

Maunuksela, E.-L. (1993) Nonsteroidal anti-inflammatory drugs in pediatric pain management. In: Schechter,N.L., Berde, C.B. and Yaster, M. (eds), *Pain in Infants, Children, and Adolescents*. Williams & Wilkins, Baltimore, pp. 135–143.

McCaffery, M. (1977) Pain relief for the child. *Pediatric Nursing*, **3**(4): 11–16.

McGrath, P.J. and Unruh, A. (1987) *Pain in Children and Adolescents*. Elsevier, Amsterdam.

McQuay, H.J. (1992) The relief of pain. In: Grahame-Smith, D.G. and Aronson, J.K. (eds), *Oxford Textbook of Clinical Pharmacology and Drug Therapy*. Oxford University Press, Oxford, pp. 458–464.

Miser, A.W., Davis, D.M., Hughs, C.S., Mulne, A.F. and Miser, J.S. (1983) Continuous subcutaneous infusion of morphine in children with cancer. *American Journal of Diseases in Children*, **137**: 383–385.

Morton, N. (1993) Balanced analgesia for children. *Nursing Standard Supplement*, **7**(25): 8–10.

Okkola, K., Maunnksela, E.L., Korpela, R. and Rosenberg, P.H. (1988) Kinetics and dynamics of postoperative intravenous morphine in children. *Clinical Pharmacology and Therapeutics*, **44**: 128–136.

Page, G.G. (1991) Chronic pain and the child with juvenile rheumatoid arthritis. *Journal of Pediatric Health Care*, **5**(1): 18–23.

Panfilli, R., Brunckhorst, L. and Dundon, R. (1988) Nursing implications of patient-controlled analgesia. *Journal of Intravenous Nursing*, **11**(2): 75–77.

Price, S. (1991) Student nurses and children's pain. *Nursing Standard*, **5**(29): 25–28.

Price, S. (1992) Student nurses' assessment of children in pain. *Journal of Advanced Nursing*, **17**: 441–447.

Rauen, K.H. and Ho, M. (1989) Children's use of patient controlled analgesia after spine surgery. *Pediatric Nursing*, **15**(6): 589–593.

Rodgers, B.M., Webb, C.J., Stergois, D. *et al.* (1988) Patient-controlled analgesia in pediatric surgery. *Journal of Pediatric Surgery*, **23**: 259–262.

Roop Moyer, S.M. and Howe, C.J. (1991) Pediatric pain intervention in the PACU. *Critical Care Nursing Clinics of North America*, **3**(1): 49–57.

Sartori, P.C.E., Gordon, G.J. and Darbyshire, P.J. (1990) Continuous papaveretum infusion for control of pain in painful sickling crisis. *Archives of Disease in Childhood*, **65**: 1151–1153.

Schechter, N., Allen, D.A. and Hanson, K. (1986) Status of pediatric pain control: a comparison of hospital analgesic use in children and adults. *Pediatrics*, **77**(1): 11–15.

Schechter, N., Berrien, F. and Shoshana, M. (1988) PCA for adolescents in sickle cell crisis. *American Journal of Nursing*, **88**(5): 719–722.

Schechter, N.L., Weisman, S.J., Rosenblum, M., Beck, A., Altman, A., Quinn, J. and Conrad, P.F. (1990) Sedation for pain procedures in children with cancer using the fentanyl lollipop: a preliminary report. In: Tyler, D.C. and Krane, E.J. (eds), *Advances in Pain Research Therapy*, Vol. 15. Raven Press, New York, pp. 209–214.

Sethna, N.F. and Wilder, R.T. (1993) Regional anesthetic techniques for chronic pain. In: Schechter, N.L., Berde, C.B. and Yaster, M. (eds), *Pain in Infants, Children and Adolescents*. Williams & Wilkins, Baltimore, pp. 281–293.

Wahstedt, C., Kollberg, G., Solh, H., Greenberg, M. and deVeber, L. (1987) Lignocaine–Prilocaine cream reduces venepuncture pain. *Lancet*, 106.

Wates, L. (1992) Pharmacologic strategies for managing pain in children. *Orthopedic Nursing*, **11**(1): 34–40.

Webb, C.J., Stergois, D.A. and Rodgers, B.M. (1989) Patient-controlled analgesia as postoperative pain treatment for children. *Journal of Pediatric Nursing*, **4**(3): 151–159.

Whaley, L.F. and Wong, D.L. (1991) *Nursing Care of Infants and Children*. Mosby–Year Book, St Louis.

Williams, J. (1987) Managing paediatric pain. *Nursing Times*, **83**(36): 36–39.

Williamson, P.S. and Williamson, M.L. (1983) Physiologic stress reduction by local anesthetic during newborn circumcision. *Pediatrics*, **71**(1): 36–40.

Woolf, C.J. (1989) Recent advances in the pathophysiology of acute pain. *British Journal of Anaesthesia*, **63**: 139–146.

Yaster, M. (1987) Analgesia and anesthesia in neonates. *Journal of Pediatrics*, **111**: 394–395.

Yaster, M. and Deshpande, J.K. (1988) Management of pediatric pain with opioid analgesics. *Journal of Pediatrics*, **113**(3): 421–429.

Yaster, M. and Maxwell, L.G. (1989) Pediatric regional analgesia. *Anesthesiology*, **70**: 324–338.

Yaster, M. and Maxwell, L.G. (1993) Opioid agonists and antagonists. In: Schechter, N.L., Berde, C.B. and Yaster, M. (eds), *Pain in Infants, Children and Adolescents*. Williams & Wilkins, Baltimore, pp. 145–171.

Yaster, M. (1990) Midazolam–fentanyl intravenous sedation in children: case report of respiratory arrest. *Pediatrics*, **86**(3): 463–467.

Holistic/therapeutic nursing care | 5

INTRODUCTION

There are a wide range of non-pharmacologically based techniques for helping to manage a child's pain. These care strategies or techniques provide a rich ground for developing holistic care, spending time with the child and working in partnership with the child and their family. These approaches to the management of pain are diverse and sometimes difficult to define under a single heading – but they can all be part of a holistic, therapeutic approach to nursing the child. Many of the techniques can be taught or facilitated by nurses so that the child and/or their family can take over this aspect of their pain management. Despite the great rewards that can be achieved by using a variety of approaches in pain management the nurse must be aware of their responsibility to deliver safe and competent care to the child and their family. This means that the nurse must ensure that they have acquired the appropriate skills, knowledge and level of competence in respect to the differing strategies and that these strategies are supported by local policies. Accredited courses can be undertaken in therapies such as massage and aromatherapy and many 'in-house' courses are offered to ensure that the nurse has achieved an appropriate standard of practice in some of the other therapies. The introduction of standards of care for monitoring the usage of the various therapeutic approaches should be carefully considered. Nurses should not implement or be encouraged to implement practices that they are not prepared for but should be encouraged to develop and enhance their therapeutic skills and thus enhance their scope of practice. McMahon (1991) sees nursing as therapy and states that:

> Therapeutic nursing, then, is about promoting health and healing for clients under their care. This healing is not 'in spite of' the nursing care, but as a direct result of deliberate nurse decision making. (p. 3).

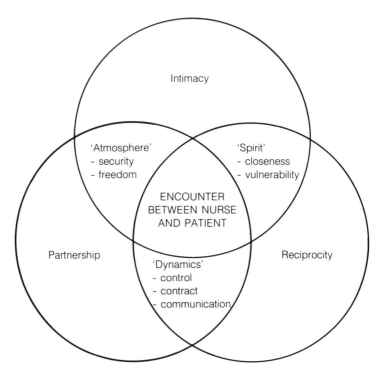

Figure 5.1 Muetzel's model of activities and factors in the therapeutic relationship.

The scope for positive 'deliberate nursing decisions' is wide in the field of pain management. Six activities underpin therapeutic nursing; these reflect a belief in holism as a concept. Muetzel (1988) sees that the therapeutic encounter with a patient is based on, and linked by, the three concepts of partnership, intimacy and reciprocity. The concepts of atmosphere, spirit and dynamics link these concepts (Fig. 5.1).

Partnership implies a relationship in which both parties gain; intimacy refers to a closeness between the two people that is of value; and reciprocity refers to the idea that the nurse can receive information and care and co-operation (Muetzel, 1988; McMahon, 1991). All of these concepts are crucial elements in the effective management and care of children and their families, particularly so in respect to their pain. By keeping these key concepts in mind when caring for the child the nurse should be able to provide a firm basis for successful nursing intervention. Nurses should and must make 'deliberate nursing decisions' with the child and their family, where appropriate, in order to help them to manage their pain. These deliberate actions in using a range of additional measures provide the best opportunity to manage the multidimensional experience of pain. McCaffery and Wong (1993) see that non-pharmacological approaches may well be the province of the nurse, as they could otherwise be overlooked. However, they warn that two precautions should be heeded:

1. Non pharamcological methods of pain control are probably most effective as coping strategies, not for actual reduction of the intensity of pain. Although there are some exceptions to this statement, such as in the use of cold, the most likely outcome of techniques such as relaxation and distraction is that pain will be more tolerable, not necessarily less severe in intensity.

2. Non pharmacologic methods of pain control may be overused or even abused with certain children or in selected circumstances. Children who are cooperative and adept at techniques such as distraction may actually suffer in silence and not be provided with appropriate analgesia or local anesthesia. (p. 312).

These precautions are worth keeping in mind as they focus the responsibility on the nurse for ensuring that non-pharmacological/therapeutic nursing

Table 5.1 Comparison of relaxation, imagery and hypnosis (reproduced with permission from Zahourek, *Relaxation and Imagery: Tools for Therapeutic Communication and Intervention*; published by W.B. Saunders Co., 1988)

Relaxation therapy	Guided imagery	Hypnosis–trance
Muscle and/or physiologically oriented	Mentally and/or imaginatively oriented	Muscles, mental or both
Directive in approach	Direct or indirect	Direct or indirect
Involves patient's trying	Usually involves the patient's trying	May or may not involve patient's trying
Expectation of specific physical results	May or may not be geared to specific expectations of mental process	May or may not involve specific results
Alters physiological processes	Usually alters physiological processes	Usually alters physiological processes
May alter mental processes	Usually alters mental processes	Usually alters mental processes
May stimulate imagery	May stimulate relaxation	May stimulate relaxation and/or imagery
Provides mental distraction	Provides mental distraction	Provides mental distraction
May promote creative thinking	Promotes creative thinking	Promotes creative thinking
May use direct suggestion of comfort and relaxation	Usually uses direct suggestion of comfort associated with a specific image	May use direct or indirect suggestions for comfort
May be used to promote healing	May be used to promote healing	May be used to promote healing

approaches are not imposed on an unwilling child and that the expectation of the child, family and the nurse are realistic. The nurse should also be aware that if the technique requires some level of input from the child this may be beyond them at times if they feel very tired or simply in too much pain to try and learn the technique (Cleeland, 1986). Additionally these strategies should, whenever possible, be introduced to the child prior to any experience of pain. Every technique that is used has its own special characteristics to offer and some of the techniques may be more readily accepted by the health professional and the child and their family. Nurses should, however, be prepared to adopt a problem/need-solving approach in respect to pain and to develop their existing skills. Despite the wide range of interventions possible nurses must ensure that they become equally skilled and knowledgeable in respect to the seemingly simple comfort measures which are a vital part of their role in pain management. Good positioning, adequate support to limbs and effective mouth care are just a small part of the nursing care that the nurse must deliver as part of their pain management strategy and they should never be overlooked in a dash to use another approach. Holistic care involves ensuring that the child's basic needs are attended to. Basic nursing care perhaps implies that anybody can carry out the care but careful positioning of the child to minimize pain, for example, takes skill, experience and a degree of intuition. Providing an optimum environment for the child is seen by Barkin (1989) to be a crucial part of their management. Barkin (1989) proposes that a good environment needs to be safe and secure, with the child's parents present, with a decrease in extraneous noise and activities and a supportive positive attitude engendered by the staff.

Three beneficial approaches to the management of pain are relaxation, imagery and hypnosis, and Zahourek (1988) provides a comparison of relaxation, imagery and hypnosis which is useful for the uninitiated (Table 5.1).

DISTRACTION

Distraction is a means of putting pain at the 'periphery of awareness' (McCaffery, 1990) and focusing attention on something other than the pain itself. Children tend to be 'especially talented' at this means of pain relief (McCaffery and Beebe, 1989). Many distractors can be used with children, including play (active or quiet), having stories read to them (especially pop-up picture books for younger children), singing and tapping the rhythms of songs and stories via headphones (active listening like this provides a strong distractor), looking at pictures, watching a favourite television programme or video, using humour (such as telling jokes), and encouraging the child to concentrate on yelling and shouting out (something appropriate to the child such as 'ouch') (McCaffery and Beebe, 1989; McCaffery, 1990; Whaley and Wong, 1991; McCaffery and Wong, 1993). The distractors can be turned up or down as the pain gets worse or better; for example, the child can sing louder or softer, shout louder or softer, turn their music up or down, tap more heavily and so on.

Table 5.2 Characteristics of effective distraction strategies for brief episodes of pain (reproduced with permission from McCaffery and Beebe, *Pain: Clinical Manual for Nursing Practice*; published by Mosby-Year Book Inc., St Louis, 1989)

1. Interesting to the patient
2. Consistent with patient's energy level and ability to concentrate
3. Rhythm is included and emphasized, e.g. keeping time to music
4. Stimulates the major sensory modalities:
   Hearing
   Vision
   Touch
   Movement
5. Capable of providing a change in stimuli when the pain changes,
   e.g. ↑ stimuli for ↑ pain

Distraction appears to be best in helping the child to deal with relatively short-duration pain such as with procedural pain. Fowler-Kerry and Ramsay-Lander (1990) report that older children benefited more from distraction techniques than the younger children in their study although they suggest that the distractors used in the study (music and lyrics) would have perhaps been more appropriate for the older children. The distractors that are chosen should be chosen in partnership with the child and their family and the technique should be introduced to the child well in advance of the pain. The techniques chosen should be well within the child's physical abilities in terms of energy levels and physical constraints. Children successfully utilizing distraction may not look like they are in pain – even though distraction does not make the pain go away. This must be taken on board by those caring for the child, as the child's perception of the pain will return once the distraction is over. McCaffery and Beebe (1989) propose characteristics of effective distraction techniques that should be considered when using this approach for the management of short-duration pain (Table 5.2).

RELAXATION

Relaxation provides relief or reduction from anxiety and a decrease in skeletal muscular tension, and whilst it does not actually reduce the child's pain it can decrease some of the distress associated with the pain experienced. Weisenberg (1980) suggests that since a person cannot be relaxed and anxious concurrently pain tolerance should be increased if the person is relaxed. Muscle pain can heighten painful stimuli; indeed the gate control theory predicts that a decrease in muscle tension will reduce pain sensation even if there is no muscle-related aetiology. Relaxation is a means by which the child can cope with pain and appropriate strategies include deep breathing, slow, rhythmic breathing, blowing away imaginary feathers, tightly squeezing their mother's hand and then slowly relaxing their grip; blowing bubbles and progressive relaxation (McCaffery and Beebe, 1989; May 1992; Whaley and Wong, 1991; Kuttner, 1986). May (1992) states that:

> a relaxed body will cope with pain and anxiety better, and that both will be reduced if the child is able to focus on something other than the procedure. (p. 27)

Relaxation provides physiological benefits, including a decrease in respiratory rate and oxygen consumption. Heart rate is often reduced and blood pressure can be lowered if the child is hypertensive. An increase in alpha waves is also reported as well as a decrease in skeletal muscular tension (Benson *et al.*, 1974; Benson, 1975; Titlebaum, 1988; Kitzinger, 1979). James (1992) proposes that cortical arousal, sympathetic nervous system activation and muscle tension are all closely related, are relevant to chronic pain and amenable to relaxation. An increase in one is liable to cause an increase in the others.

Relaxation can help with sleep and this is important, as fatigue or exhaustion can make pain much more difficult to cope with (Diamond and Coniam, 1991). Additionally relaxation can reduce tension, a stressor, and provide a level of mental calm. Some people may experience a feeling of warmth, usually focused in the stomach, during relaxation (James, 1992). Relaxation is particularly appropriate for the management of chronic pain, where it can be used to help control pain levels and prevent them from becoming too intense. Douglas (1993) suggests that children under the age of 7 years can be helped to achieve a relaxed state by being asked to become floppy like a rag doll. Progressive muscle relaxation is a technique that children can adopt quite readily. With progressive relaxation the child is encouraged to adopt a comfortable position and then told to progressively make their body go limp and heavy, starting with their toes. Children often prefer to have their eyes open when they are relaxing.

Young children and infants enjoy and benefit from the relaxation that can result from their parents gently rocking them or stroking them in a rhythmic manner. Infants often display disorganized and jittery movements in response to pain, and rocking and comforting the baby can help them to establish a level of organization and this can result in a reduction in stress (Roop Moyer and Howe, 1991). Infants also appreciate being able to feel the boundaries of their environment by being cradled within a 'nest' of blankets which can provide a degree of security (D'Apolita, 1985).

Relaxation can be used by children as a self-help approach. Engel (1992) reports the use of progressive relaxation in the management of recurrent, non-malignant headaches in children. The study showed an increase in the number of headache-free days once the child had adopted this strategy. Migraine headache in children was the focus of studies by Masek *et al.* (1984) and Richter *et al.* (1986), and relaxation training was found to be of value. Sokel *et al.* (1991) report that children experiencing recalcitrant abdominal pain who used a variety of pain control techniques including relaxation were able to remove or reduce their pain so that they were able to resume normal activities. Children were able to develop a sense of control over their pain and were able to 'save face' and 'maintain dignity'.

IMAGERY

Imagery is the use of imagination to modify the response to pain (Doody *et al.*, 1991). Imagery involves using sensory images that modify the pain to make it more bearable or to substitute a pleasant image in place of pain. Dossey *et al.* (1984) cited in Doody *et al.* (1991) state that imagery 'provides a focus and organized energy to facilitate healing'.

Imagery provides relief through distraction, relaxation and producing an image of pain. Imagery can be used in a guided way so that the child imagines something about their pain that will help to reduce it. This deliberate and systematic approach is generally discussed as guided therapeutic imagery. Normally pleasant images are pictured that perhaps 'remedy' the pain and distress being experienced; for example, a child who is hot could imagine a cool environment, or if the child has pain the pain can be pictured flowing out of their body. Children can also use imagery to imagine their analgesics and other drugs going around their body to the place where their pain is and taking it away. The child may also imagine themselves as being their favourite character from the television or books, and so on. Playing out the role of their hero figure can help them with managing their pain. Children may also appreciate becoming involved in a story that is read or played to them when they have pain and being asked questions about what happens next, and other questions fired by the child's active involvement in the story (McCaffery and Beebe, 1989; Kuttner, 1986; Doody *et al.*, 1991).

Children may also respond to the concept of the healing ball of light or energy. This imaginary ball of energy becomes the focus of the child's attention and the energy from the ball travels to the affected painful areas, where it absorbs the pain and takes it away (McCaffery and Beebe, 1989). Imagery can help the child to confront and modify their pain, thus taking some level of control over it.

MASSAGE

Massage is the systematic manual manipulation of the soft tissues of the body to produce relaxation of the muscles; it promotes circulation of the blood and lymph, relief from pain, restoration of metabolic balance as well as other physical and emotional benefits (Beck, 1988). It is an ancient method of maintaining and improving health. Massage is not only healing in its own right but the level of contact achieved through massage is a vital component of the therapy (Tisserand, 1977). Massage has effects on the muscular, physiological, nervous and circulatory systems. Additionally it has well-established psychological effects and enhances the feeling of well-being. Children may benefit from the use of a gentle relaxing massage either to the whole body or to part of the body. Obviously, as with all forms of treatment, the child should be involved in the decision-making process and should, wherever appropriate give their permission. Massage provides healing and relaxes tight contracted muscles that are perhaps the result of pain-induced stress. Massage and the sense of relaxation it engenders is often followed by a period of renewed energy (Davis, 1988). This can be important if the child feels very tired as a result of dealing with their pain. At one level massage acts as a form of cutaneous stimulation which may in itself modify the pain experience by stimulating the large-diameter nerve fibres responsible for inhibiting pain perception by 'closing the gate' and perhaps through stimulating the production of endogenous endorphins (McCaffery and Beebe, 1989). However, the feeling of relaxation that can be created and the opportunity to modify or relieve pain are aims which can be achieved by using massage. The nurse can actively involve the child's family in learning how to perform the massage and so become more involved in their child's care.

TOUCH

Touch is a two-way process involving both sensation and cognition. The need to be touched is present at birth and it is a continuing and developing need. Touch provides one of the strongest means of communicating caring and empathy. Many children despite being cared for in loving hospital environments are deprived of affective and therapeutic touch – even though they are at risk from a high level of instrumental touch. Blackburn and Barnard (1985) showed that the mean number of loving touches in a neonatal unit was about five touches per 24 hours. Mitchell (1985) found that staff other than the nurses rarely touched the patients except to do physical examination and that the nurses themselves most often touched the children when they were performing procedures. The parents, especially those of the most severely ill children, touched more often than the nurses. This study, which focused on intracranial pressure measurement, demonstrated that touch alone (not related to procedures) never raised intracranial pressure beyond an individual's own physiological variability.

Touch can be seen to be a vital means of communicating empathy, care and concern for the child and their pain (Day, 1995). Touch can be provided through both affective touch – which is generally seen to be caring, loving touch – and therapeutic touch, which aims to be healing, such as in the Krieger--Kunz technique or the laying on of hands (Wright, 1987).

Therapeutic touch

Therapeutic touch or the laying on of hands is a form of healing that was systematically developed by Krieger in the 1970s. It has been shown in a number of studies to reduce anxiety, promote relaxation and relieve pain (Krieger, 1975; Heidt, 1981; 1990). Krieger sees healing or therapeutic touch as a nursing 'modality' and this technique is another nursing intervention in which growing interest is shown. Therapeutic touch, as developed by Krieger, follows four steps: centring, assessment, unruffling and treatment/directing energy phase. Therapeutic touch aims to treat disturbances in the child's energy field, such as those created by pain and disease, and to provide a balance in the whole field. Imbalances occur where there is pain, disease and so on. Centring is the phase in which the nurse (acting as healer) passes their hands over the child's body (about 100–150 cm away), moving from the head to the feet. The nurse picks up differences in the energy flow and these are described as areas of congestion. During the unruffling or mobilizing phase the nurse uses sweeping movements of the hands to cover the body until congestion is relieved and the energy field feels smooth. The treatment phase is when the nurse/healer redirects or channels energy to the child to rebalance their energy field where there are deficits in energy. Finally the nurse reassesses the energy field to check for a return to or towards balance. Turton (1988) reports a case study by Tinnerin, who has successfully used therapeutic touch in children to relieve inflammation.

Therapeutic touch provides another means for the nurse to help to manage the child's pain and as a non-invasive method it may have much to offer. Further research, especially in respect to what therapeutic touch can offer children, needs to be undertaken although the anecdotal evidence seems to be fairly convincing.

AROMATHERAPY

Aromatherapy is a holistic form of healing that uses essential oils extracted from aromatic plants. Although this is an ancient form of healing it is an area that has not attracted huge amounts of interest from conventional medicine until relatively recently. Aromatherapy is now being used with increasing frequency within the hospital, hospice and community setting as a means of reducing stress, relaxing, treating symptoms and providing relief from pain. It can be used as the sole means of treating pain but is often used in conjunction with other approaches. Aromatherapy oils can promote healing on different levels – physical; emotional and mental – and can be used in massage oils, in baths, through inhalations and through compresses. Aromatherapy, within the hands of a professional therapist, is a safe and potentially very effective means of reducing pain, including anxiety, sadness and fear. Aromatherapy massage engenders a feeling of security and children will often readily accept a gentle relaxing massage, especially if it smells good as well (Day, 1995). Aromatherapy massage strokes can offer several means of reducing the experience of pain and this can be done in five main ways: by acting at the trigger site; by acting on the gating mechanism; by stimulating the inhibitory control system; positively affecting the cognitive control mechanism; and by encouraging the balance of chi (energy) and the release of endorphins and dynorphins.

Children can be successfully treated with diluted essential oils. It is recommended that a 1–2% dilution of oils is used for children (Davis, 1988). Perhaps the most commonly used oil for children is camomile, which has good relaxing, soothing properties as well as anti-inflammatory properties. *Matricaria chamomilla* (German camomile) is a particularly effective anti-inflammatory oil owing to the presence of azulene (an anti-inflammatory agent). Lavender oil is another oil that can generally be used with safety with young children; lavender has analgesic, sedating and calming properties and it is very good to use on skin that is inflamed or burned. For babies a drop of lavender oil (*Lavandula angustifolia*) and camomile (*Matricaria chamomilla* or *Anthemis nobilis*) mixed well with a few teaspoons of a carrier oil such as sweet almond oil can be added to their bath to help relax them and soothe their pain. Alternatively a gentle massage using lavender or camomile mixed with a carrier oil can be very soothing for both the infant and the parents. Older children may benefit from the use of peppermint (*Mentha piperita*), geranium (*Pelargonium graveolens*) and rose (*Rosa centifolia*) along with the use of lavender and camomile. These oils have a variety of properties but rose and geranium are excellent at calming the child who is anxious with their pain and encouraging them to relax (Davis, 1988; Tisserand, 1977; Worwood, 1990). When the oils are burned they may facilitate the child's use of other strategies such as imagery.

Aromatherapy should only ever be practised by a trained practitioner, although once the oils have been made into a safe and effective blend the parents and other nurses should be encouraged to use them within the 'regime' chosen by the therapist.

TRANSCUTANEOUS ELECTRICAL NERVE STIMULATION

Transcutaneous electrical nerve stimulation (TENS) as a management strategy for children is a somewhat unknown quantity since very few research studies have been published and it appears to be a relatively underused approach (Eland, 1993; Lander and Fowler-Kerry, 1993). TENS aims to relieve pain and is a non-invasive, safe method to use (Lander and Fowler-Kerry, 1993). The TENS device delivers controlled, low-voltage electricity to the body via electrodes (two or more may be used) placed on the skin. Two major forms of TENS are generally used: (a) continuous TENS (a continuous flow of pulses at a preset frequency; and (b) 'burst' or pulsed TENS ('intermittent trains at about 2 Hz of pulses at a preset frequency') (Thompson, 1992). TENS is useful in localized pain and it is thought to increase endorphin levels (burst TENS) and perhaps to act as a counter-irritant (McCaffery and Beebe, 1989). The TENS recipient will often describe a sensation of tingling when the device is working.

The studies available in relation to the use of TENS with children provide a clue to the potential value of TENS (Carmen and Roach, 1988; Finley and Steward, 1983) but because of some problems with the validity of the studies they do not provide real evidence.

Lander and Fowler-Kerry (1993) in a study of children aged 5–17 years, using TENS as a means of pain reduction associated with venepuncture, found that the children in the TENS treatment group had lower pain scores than those in the placebo TENS group and the control group (even though the effect was small). The children appeared to tolerate and accept TENS well. The youngest children (aged 5–7 years) experienced/reported the worse pain. Lander and Fowler-Kerry conclude that TENS requires further investigation but that it may have a place in the management of children's pain.

Eland (1993) presents a series of seven case studies on children aged 4–17 years experiencing pain from a variety of medical and surgical problems who used TENS to successfully manage pain associated with amphotericin infusion, phantom limb, neuroblastoma and others. The TENS electrodes, where appropriate, were placed over acupuncture points and controlled pain of both short- and longer-term duration.

TENS would therefore seem to have a future as one of the non-invasive, child-accepted strategies for managing pain.

ACUPUNCTURE

Acupuncture is a system of ancient medicine, healing and Eastern philosophy (Mann 1992a, 1992b) originating in China 8000–3000 years BC. Acupuncture aims to redress imbalances of Yin and Yang through balancing the flow of Qi (ch'i or energy) by inserting acupuncture needles into specific points along the 14 meridians (Steel, 1988). Acupuncture aims to allow the body to heal itself; it is a holistic treatment inasmuch as it treats the person, not the disease or symptoms (Downey, 1988). Acupuncture, whilst it has a well-respected and long-established history in the East, has not yet been explained using a Western, biomedical, scientific approach and this has resulted in its being regarded with a degree of suspicion. However, studies suggest that acupuncture encourages the production of endorphins (He, 1987). Pomeranz (1987) suggests that acupuncture stimulates the production of endorphins, promotes central analgesia and has inhibitory effects on the pain pathway. Studies on the use of acupuncture in children are exceptionally limited although it is reported to be used successfully in a range of children's illnesses (Caborn, 1988). Caborn (1988) reports that despite children's normal reluctance to have anything to do with needles:

> Not only do children respond very quickly to acupuncture but the slender needles are a great deal less daunting to them than many items of traditional medical equipment. (p. 31).

Yee *et al.* (1993) confirm the lack of research studies associated with acupuncture and children's acute or chronic pain and conclude it is therefore problematic to draw definitive conclusions about the role that acupuncture has to play.

HYPNOSIS

Hypnosis has been found to be of value in the care and management of children with both acute and chronic pain. Hypnosis can be defined, according to Valente (1991), as:

> focused attention, an altered state of consciousness, or a trance, often accompanied by relaxation. (p. 699)

and a state in which 'the subject becomes receptive to suggestions' (Tyrer, 1992). Hypnosis is useful in relieving distress and pain and in improving a child's self-confidence (LaBaw and Holton, 1975; Olness and Gardner, 1988). Hilgard and LeBaron (1984) report the successful use of hypnosis in children with cancer, and Zelter and LeBaron (1982) found it more effective in reducing the pain associated with bone marrow aspirations than distraction and self-control techniques. Children can be induced into an altered state of awareness through the use of play, imagery and relaxation and they are generally very good subjects. Children can use their vivid imaginations during the trance to picture a positive and interesting experience involving their favourite hero or heroine, their favourite place or memory. The child's own toys and their favourite music and so on can be used to make the experience real (Kuttner, 1989). Valente (1991) reports that one session or trance is often sufficient to prepare a child for a bone marrow aspiration or lumbar puncture under hypnosis, although some children may need two to four practice sessions. Children can also learn self-hypnosis, which allows them greater freedom to manage or control their painful experiences (LaBaw and Holton, 1975; Olness and Gardner, 1988). Valente (1991) proposes three stages for hypnosis pain relief:

> (1) inducing and deepening the trance; (2) suggesting pain relief; and (3) ending the trance. (p. 702)

Kuttner (1993) suggests that although the child's vivid imagination is one of their biggest assets in respect to hypnotherapy it also places a demand on the clinician to be flexible and able to enter the child's imaginary world in order for the treatment to be successful.

Hypnosis does not actually take the pain away but it decreases/removes the child's perception of it. Woods (1989) proposes that hypnosis stimulates the higher centres of the brain so that they inhibit the opening of the gate.

Again this therapy requires further investigation although it has been used quite widely in the USA, especially within the care of children with cancer.

REFERENCES

Barkin, R.M. (1989) Analgesia for children: options and choices. *Annals of Emergency Medicine*, **18**(5): 592/151–152/593.

Beck, M. (1988) *The Theory and Practice of Therapeutic Massage*. Milady, New York.

Benson, H. (1975) *The Relaxation Response*. William Morrow, New York.

Benson, H., Beery, J.F. and Carol, M.P. (1974) The relaxation response. *Psychiatry*, **37**: 37–46.

Blackburn, S. and Barnard, K.E. (1985) Analysis of care giving events in preterm infants in the special care unit. In: Gottfried, A.W. and Gaiter, I. (eds), *Infant Stress under Intensive Care*. University Park Press. Baltimore, pp. 113–129.

Caborn, A. (1988) Point taken. *Nursing Times*, **84**(10): 31–33.

Carmen, D. and Roach, J. (1988) Transcutaneous electrical nerve stimulation for the relief of post operative pain in children. *Spine*, **13**: 109–110.

Cleeland, C. (1986) Behavioral control of symptoms. *Journal of Pain and Symptom Management*, **1**(1): 36–38.

D'Apolita, K. (1984) The neonate's response to pain II. *Maternal Child Nursing*, **9**: 256–257.

Davis, P. (1988) *Aromatherapy: An A–Z*. CW Daniel, Saffron Walden.

Day, S. (1995) Complementary therapies. In: Carter, B. and Dearmun, A.K. (eds) *Child Health Care Nursing: Concepts, Theory and Practice*. Blackwell Scientific Publications, Oxford. (In press)

Diamond, A.W. and Coniam, S.W. (1991) *The Management of Chronic Pain*. Oxford University Press, Oxford.

Doody, S.B., Smith, C., Webb, J. (1991) Nonpharmacologic interventions for pain management. *Critical Care Nursing Clinics of North America*, **3**(1): 69–75.

Dossey, B.M. and Gruzzetta, C.E. (1984) *Cardiovascular Nursing Body Mind Tapestry*. C.V. Mosby, St. Louis.

Douglas, J. (1993) *Psychology and Nursing Children*. Macmillan/British Psychological Society, Leicester.

Downey, S. (1988) Acupuncture. In: Rankin-Box, D.F. (ed.) *Complementary Health Therapies: A Guide for Nurses and the Caring Professions*. Croom Helm, London, pp. 8–26.

Eland, J. (1993) The use of TENS with children. In: Schechter, N.L., Berde, C.B. and Yaster, M. (eds), *Pain in Infants, Children, and Adolescents*. Williams & Wilkins, Baltimore, pp. 331–339.

Engel, J.M. (1992) Relaxation training: a self-help approach for children with headaches. *American Journal of Occupational Therapy*, **46**(7): 591–596.

Finley, G. and Steward, D. (1983) Transcutaneous electric nerve stimulation for control of postoperative pain following spinal fusion in adolescents. *Canadian Anesthetists Society Journal*, **30**: 67.

Fowler-Kerry and Ramsay-Lander, J. (1990) Utilizing cognitive strategies to relieve pain in young children. In: Tyler, D.C. and Krane, E.J. (eds), *Advances in Pain Research Therapy*, Vol. 15. Raven Press, New York, pp. 247–253.

He, L. (1987) Involvement of endogenous opioid peptides in acupuncture analgesia. *Pain*, **31**: 99–121.

Heidt, P.R. (1981) Effects of therapeutic touch on anxiety levels of hospitalised patients. *Nursing Research*, **30**(1): 32–37.

Heidt, P.R. (1990) Openness: a qualitative analysis of nurses' and patients' experiences of therapeutic touch. *IMAGE: Journal of Nursing Scholarship*, **22**: 180–186.

Hilgard, J. and LeBaron, S. (1984) *Hypnotherapy of Pain in Children with Cancer*. W. Kaufman, Los Altos, CA.

James, P.T. (1992) Use of relaxation. In: Tyrer, S.P. (ed.), *Psychology, Psychiatry, and Chronic Pain*. Butterworth Heinemann, Oxford, pp. 119–135.

Kitzinger, S. (1979) *Birth at Home*. Oxford University Press, New York.

Krieger, D. (1975) Therapeutic touch: the imprimatur of nursing. *American Journal of Nursing*, **75**(5): 784–787.

Kuttner, L. (1986) *No Fears, no Tears: Children with Cancer Coping with Pain*. Canadian Cancer Society, Vancouver, BC.

Kuttner, L. (1989) Management of young children's acute pain and anxiety during invasive medical procedures. *Pediatrician*, **16**: 39–44.

Kuttner, L. (1993) Hypnotic interventions for children in pain. In: Schechter, N.L., Berde, C.B. and Yaster, M. (eds), *Pain in Infants, Children, and Adolescents*. Williams & Wilkins, Baltimore, pp. 229–236

LaBaw, W.C. and Holton, C. (1975) Use of self-hypnosis in children with cancer. *American Journal of Clinical Hypnosis*, **17**(4): 233–238.

Lander, J. and Fowler-Kerry, S. (1993) TENS for children's procedural pain. *Pain*, **52**: 209–216.

Mann, F. (1992a) *Acupuncture: Cure of Many Diseases*, 2nd edn. Butterworth Heinemann, Oxford.

Mann, F. (1992b) *Reinventing Acupuncture: A New Concept of Ancient Medicine*. Butterworth Heinemann, Oxford.

Masek, B., Russo, D. and Varni, J. (1984) Behavioral approaches to the management of chronic pain in children. *Pediatric clinics of North America*, **31**: 1113–1131.

May, L. (1992) Reducing pain and anxiety in children. *Nursing Standard*, **6**(44): 25–28.

McCaffery, M. (1990) Nursing approaches to nonpharmacological pain control. *International Journal of Nursing Studies*, **27**(1): 1–5.

McCaffery, M. and Beebe, A. (1989) *Pain Clinical Manual for Nursing Practice*. Mosby, St Louis.

McCaffery, M. and Wong, D.L. (1993) Nursing interventions for pain control in children In: Schechter, N.L., Berde, C.B. and Yaster, M. (eds), *Pain in Infants, Children, and Adolescents.* Williams & Wilkins, Baltimore, pp. 295–316.

McMahon, R. (1991) Therapeutic nursing: theory, issues and practice. In: McMahon, R. and Pearson, A. (eds), *Nursing as Therapy.* Chapman & Hall, London, pp. 1–25.

Mitchell, P. (1985) Critically ill children: the importance of touch in a high technological environment. *Nursing Administration Quarterly,* **9**(4): 38–46.

Muetzel, P.-A. (1988) Therapeutic nursing. In: Pearson, A. (ed.), *Primary Nursing: Nursing in the Burford and Oxford Nursing Development Units.* Chapman & Hall, London, pp. 89–116.

Olness, K. and Gardner, G. (1988) *Hypnosis and Hypnotherapy with Children.* Grune & Stratton, New York.

Pearson, A. (1991) Therapeutic nursing: theory, issues and practice. In: McMahon, R. and Pearson, A. (eds), *Nursing as Therapy.* Chapman & Hall, London, pp. 1–25.

Pomeranz, B. (1987) The scientific basis of acupuncture. In Stux, G. and Pomeranz, B. (eds), *Acupuncture.* Springer-Verlag, Berlin.

Richter, I.L., McGrath, P.J., Humphreys, P.J. *et al.* (1986) Cognitive and relaxation treatment of pediatric migraine. *Pain,* **25**: 195–203.

Roop Moyer, S.M. and Howe, C.J. (1991) Pediatric pain intervention in the PACU. *Critical Care Nursing Clinics of North America,* **3**(1): 49–57.

Sokel, B., Devane, S. and Bentovim, A. (1991) Getting better with honor: individual relaxation/self hypnosis techniques for control of recalcitrant abdominal pain in children. *Family Systems Medicine,* **9**(1): 83–91.

Steel, C. (1988) A brief guide to acupuncture and its concepts. *TECHNIC,* **71**: 4–5.

Thompson, J.W. (1992) Other treatment strategies (TENS and acupuncture). In: Tyrer, S.P. (ed.), *Psychology, Psychiatry, and Chronic Pain.* Butterworth Heinemann, Oxford, pp. 163–177.

Tisserand, R. (1977) *The Art of Aromatherapy.* Daniel, Saffron Walden.

Titlebaum, H. (1988) Relaxation. In: Zahourek, R.P. (ed.), *Relaxation and Imagery: Tools for Therapeutic Communication and Intervention.* Saunders, Philadelphia, pp. 28–52.

Turton, P. (1988) Healing: therapeutic touch. In: Rankin-Box, D.F. (ed.), *Complementary Health Therapies: A Guide for Nurses and the Caring Professions.* Croom Helm, London.

Tyrer, S.P. (1992) Hypnosis. In: Tyrer, S.P. (ed.), *Psychology, Psychiatry, and Chronic Pain.* Butterworth Heinemann, Oxford, pp. 149–155.

Valente, S.M. (1991) Using hypnosis with children for pain management. *Oncology Nursing Forum,* **18**(4): 699–704.

Weisenberg, M. (1980) Understanding pain phenomena. In Rachman, S. (ed.), *Contributions to Medical Psychology,* Vol. 2. Pergamon Press, Oxford, pp. 79–111.

Whaley, L.F. and Wong, D.L. (1991) *Nursing Care of Infants and Children,* 4th edn. Mosby-Year Book, St Louis.

Woods, M. (1989) Pain control and hypnosis. *Nursing Times,* **85**(7): 38–40.

Worwood, V.A. (1990) *The Fragrant Pharmacy: A Home and Health Care Guide to Aromatherapy and Essential Oils.* Bantam Books, Toronto.

Wright, S.M. (1987) The use of therapeutic touch in the management of pain. *Nursing Clinics of North America*, **22**: 705–714.

Yee, J.D., Lin, Y.-C., and Aubuchon, P.A. (1993) Acupuncture. In: Schechter, N.L., Berde, C.B. and Yaster, M. (eds), *Pain in Infants, Children, and Adolescents.* Williams & Wilkins, Baltimore, pp. 341–348.

Zahourek, R.P. (1988) Overview. Relaxation and imagery: Tools for therapeutic communication and intervention. In: Zahourek, R.P. (ed.), *Relaxation and Imagery: Tools for Therapeutic Communication and Intervention.* Sanders, Philadelphia, pp. 3–27.

Zelter, L.K. and LeBaron, S. (1982) Hypnosis and nonhypnotic techniques for reduction of pain and anxiety during painful procedures in children and adolescents with cancer. *Journal of Pediatrics*, **101**(6): 1032–1035.

Special pain experiences in children

INTRODUCTION

Every child's experience of pain is unique and unlike any other child's experience. However, some similarities exist in respect to the type of pain experienced. This chapter considers several 'special' situations/types of pain that children experience and attempts to examine these areas in some depth. It is acknowledged that many other areas have not been addressed – this is not an attempt to decry the importance of these areas but some level of focus is important. Some of the quotes contained in this chapter are from interviews with British children during their admission to a children's hospital.

PERIOPERATIVE PAIN

It hurt quite a bit, and it was itching and burning – and it hurts there round where those beads go into my tummy and when I came back [from theatre] the tube was hurting in my nose, you know, and the nurses didn't do nothing – they just came for a few seconds and then left me and the trolley was scary.

Faizan, aged 8 years, recovering
from genitourinary surgery

Perhaps one of the biggest hurdles in respect to postoperative recovery that many children have to face is the reluctance of medical staff to prescribe and nursing staff to administer appropriate analgesic cover. Postoperative pain assessment is sometimes described as being difficult; it is nonetheless important (Rivera, 1991). Despite the number of studies that have documented the degree of under-medication children are still at risk not only from under-medication but also from the stress associated with experiencing ineffectively managed postoperative pain (Anand and Carr, 1989; Beyer *et al.*, 1983; Mather and Mackie, 1983). This lack of proper attention to this aspect of care has led professionals, parents and support organizations and the media to question practice. Marks (1992) writing in *The Independent* highlighted the continued lack of adequate relief in the postoperative period under the heading 'Children's pain after operations "often undertreated"'. The association Action for Sick Children has also developed a leaflet called 'Children and Pain', which outlines the different types of analgesia and non-pharmacological means of managing pain that are available. Shelley (1993) reports that within a month of publication of the leaflet there had been a massive response, with over 2000 people requesting a leaflet. Obviously this is an area that needs urgent positive attention so that children are not traumatized by the pain they experience. This involves changing attitudes towards postoperative management so that outdated beliefs are no longer considered viable. Swafford and Allen (1968) stated that:

> Pediatric patients seldom need medication for the relief of pain after general surgery. They tolerate discomfort well. The child will say he does not feel well, or that he is uncomfortable or wants his parents, but often he will not relate this unhappiness to pain. (p. 133)

Since this study was published many researchers have established that children do experience discomfort and that they are under-medicated. Eland (1988) reports a study undertaken in 1973 that studied analgesic prescription and administration in children aged 5–8 years who were experiencing pain as a result of spinal fusions, severe burns and nephrectomies. Twenty five children were included in the study and 21 of these had analgesics prescribed. However, only 12 of the children received analgesia and a total of only 24 doses were administered throughout their whole admission. Eland and Anderson (1977) compared the administration of analgesia between 25 children and 18 adults. The children in the study received a total of 24 doses (4% of analgesics administered to the total population) whilst the adults received 671 doses (96% of the total population).

Beyer *et al.* (1983) compared postoperative prescriptions in 50 adults and 50 children. The children received 30% of all analgesics administered, whilst the adults received 70%. None of the adults received no medication but 12 infants/toddlers received no medication and six children were not prescribed any medication. Eland (1985a) in a study of 2000 children aged between 4 and 10 years who had undergone a major procedure found that 65% had no postoperative analgesia and 80% had no 'medico-legal' orders for medication. Mather and Mackie (1983) studied 170 postoperative children and found that 16% had no analgesia prescribed, 30% did not receive the analgesics that were ordered and 20% of the children received only non-opioid analgesics when there was a choice between opioid and non-opioid analgesia on the prescription sheet. Burokas (1985) found that 37% of patients were prescribed sub-therapeutic doses.

Schechter *et al.* (1986) found in a study of 90 adults and 90 children that despite the groups being matched for diagnosis and gender the adults received 1.5–2 times the number of analgesic doses as those received by the group of children. Children in the study were also less likely to be prescribed opioids.

Gadish *et al.* (1988) studied 38 nurses caring for postoperative children to determine information on their decision making in respect to pain management. Some interesting issues were highlighted. The educational level appeared to affect decision making, with nurses with a baccalaureate degree giving higher doses of analgesia compared with nurses with associate degrees, who tended to give mostly non-narcotic analgesics. Nurses consistently chose to administer analgesia rather than try other rarely used management strategies. Of the nurses studied 5% aimed to relieve pain completely, 63% aimed to relieve as much as possible and 24% aimed to relieve enough to make the 'patient function'. In respect to neonatal and infant pain the results were worrying, with 15.8% feeling that babies only experience pain after 1 month of age and 5.3% believing that pain does not occur until after 6 months of age. Additional findings from this study demonstrate that younger children were likely to receive less medication than older children. Nurses also felt that experience was more valuable than education and that they relied on physiological rather than non-verbal clues. This is also borne out in the findings of a small study on the perceptions and attitudes of nursing and medical staff towards neonatal pain (Carter, 1989). These studies demonstrate the need for a perioperative pain management plan to be considered and formulated so that children are not left to suffer physically and emotionally.

Postoperative pain is often linked to the child's fear of harm to their body. Alex and Ritchie (1992) studied 24 children (aged 7–11 years) who were interviewed on their third postoperative day about their interpretation of the experience. The majority of the children described a level of anxiety about their pain although five children did not describe any anxiety about postoperative pain. They were mostly concerned about 'perceived threats to body integrity and physical well being'. This anxiety included feelings of being confined by decreased mobility because of pain, being crippled by their pain, and being scared of needles. The children reported feelings of anger and sadness and of feeling exhausted. The children who generally experienced more pain postoperatively than they had expected never indicated that they had asked for analgesia and three children said that nurses did nothing. However, other children saw the nurse's presence as being helpful, caring and reassuring. The children suggested that nurses could help them more if they gave more information about the pain and were more sensitive in their assessment. Children in a study by O'Malley and McNamara (1993) expressed their reactions to surgery and pre/postoperative care through their drawings. Children's fears and feelings of insecurity were communicated effectively through their drawings even when outwardly they appeared to be dealing well with their admission. The authors suggest that drawings could be incorporated as part of an assessment tool.

The effective management of postoperative pain commences preoperatively wherever possible, and includes all members of the team liable to care for the child. Preparatory information needs to be age and development level appropriate and should be tailored to the child's own needs and concerns. Parents may well be the best people to give this information to the child although a nurse may need to be present to help with difficult questions (Douglas, 1993).

Fear plays some part in a child's apprehension about an operation and hospitalization and perhaps the best time to educate the child is well before admission (Fradd, 1986) as part of the child's everyday learning. Eiser and Hanson (1991) used a 'play hospital' set up in a primary school and studied the children's play. The children (5–8 years old) were filmed playing with the equipment provided on two occasions and showed changes in their knowledge of the equipment and role of the staff. The authors propose that this may be a useful preparatory technique and may reduce anxiety and/or help children deal with medical procedures. Children and their families need to have an optimum level of information and this can only be provided by knowledgeable and skilled staff (Gillies, 1993). Good communication is an essential element in the management of postoperative pain (Mather and Mackie, 1983). Both Melamed and Siegel (1975) and Vistainer and Wolfer (1975) report that anxiety and fear can be decreased with preoperative information about the trajectory of postoperative recovery. Preoperative visits to the anaesthetic room, theatre and recovery rooms can reduce levels of anxiety if they are handled effectively and children can be encouraged to dress up so that they can play out their role in a safe way. The child and their family can also ask questions and receive reassurance and more information about areas that are of greatest concern to them (McIlvaine, 1989). Despite being given information the child may feel ill-prepared when they return to the ward and experience unexpected sensations:

> it [site of circumcision] felt horrible . . . and bad . . . and it felt tingly and I didn't like it and it won't be better till I'm eight . . . why does it feel tingly?
>
> (Reese, aged 7 years, one
> day post circumcision)

Glasper (1991) discusses the role of the parent in the anaesthetic room and care by parent schemes as being helpful in reducing stress and anxiety. Traditionally, though, parents have not been allowed to accompany their child into recovery – this practice has been based on a somewhat dubious rationale. Glasper (1991) proposes that five factors may be used to prevent parents accompanying their child: local custom and practice; fear of an increased risk of infection; potential problems of having to cope with the parent (e.g. who faints); reduction in training experience opportunities; and concern about parents being critical of the procedure. None of these reasons seems to be based on the needs of the child and seems rather to be biased towards the needs or perceived needs of the professionals. This attitude seems to be particularly unfortunate when considering the studies that demonstrate the supportive element in parental presence (Hanallah, 1983). Glasper and Dewar (1986) surveyed paediatric anaesthetists about policies, attitudes and opinions concerning parental presence and found a lack of consensus in all areas (cited in Glasper, 1991).

The nurse has a crucial role in ensuring that the child and their family have an appropriate amount of information before the operation and that any concerns are allayed. Children who wish to be accompanied by their parents should be given the opportunity for this level of reassurance whenever possible. Part of the preoperative preparation of a child should be the use of EMLA (eutectic mixture of local anaesthetics), where appropriate, in preparing for the siting of an intravenous cannula. This again is important in decreasing the overall potential for pain, although as one child pointed out:

> It hurts my arms when they [nurses] take the EMLA off but now they shave my arms 'cos I've got hairy arms and it's better now – I don't like them pulling out the hairs – it hurts.
>
> (Faizan, aged 8 years)

Premedications, when required, should not be given intramuscularly as this is a known major stressor for the child and is a poor preparation for the subsequent surgery or procedure (Eland, 1985b). Premedication may be a requirement of the surgery: atropine may be required as a premedication for the infant owing to the small size of their airways. Premedications were seen to be generally necessary for invasive procedures in a survey undertaken by Klein (1992). McIlvaine (1989) states that the goal of premedication is:

> to provide perioperative sedation and analgesia, to minimize secretions, to maximize hemodynamic stability during induction and to make the induction experience more tolerable for all concerned. (p. 218).

However, Wark (1991) suggests that some anaesthetists believe that premedication may not be required once trust and rapport are established at the preoperative visit. Premedications depend on the child, the type of operative procedure and the preference of the anaesthetist, and can be given orally, intramuscularly, intravenously and rectally. The intramuscular and rectal route tend to be avoided as they are very invasive for a child. Wark (1991) divides premedications into three classes: analgesics (used for sedative and euphoric effects, such as papaveretum and pethidine); sedatives (generally given orally and including drugs such as temazepam, diazepam and trimeprazine); and the anticholinergics (used to reduce excess secretions and reduce the risk from active vagal reflexes, including drugs such as atropine and hyoscine).

Pain in the postoperative period is problematic as it may increase the potential for postoperative morbidity and mortality. Perioperative pain management by the use of regional anaesthesia as an adjunct to general anaesthesia is reported to decrease surgical stimulation of the site of the operation and this reduces the need for 'volatile and opioid agents'. Children recover more quickly from the general anaesthetic since there is a decrease in cardiovascular and respiratory depression and postoperative sedation (Benham and Murray, 1993). Dalens (1993) reports that good management of postoperative pain (resulting primarily from injured tissue) lies in preventing it and that 'regional blockade does this better than any other mode of therapy' (p. 266). Children with poorly controlled pain may be reluctant to take deep breaths and potential respiratory problems compounded by pain need to be considered. The child may suppress coughing due to muscle splinting. The child who is in pain will often be reluctant to mobilize and this may also lead to stasis of secretions. Children and infants will also experience a stress response to the surgery and the additional stressor of pain can add to the severity of this response. A hyperdynamic catabolic response may result and surgical stress has been shown to delay healing and the repair of tissues.

'Stress hormones' (corticosteroids, growth hormones, glucagon and catecholamines) are released as a result of surgery, and the use of good intraoperative techniques has been shown to reduce the levels of these stress hormones (Anand et al., 1987; Williamson and Williamson, 1983). The catabolic stress response may delay healing and recovery after surgery (Anand and Carr, 1989; Roop Moyer and Howe, 1991).

However, Cohen (1993) proposes that although the control of stress postoperatively may be beneficial:

> the alleviation of pain often has little influence in the modification of this protective reflexive response. The relief of pain and the modifica- tion of postoperative stress need separate consideration when planning and implementing post operative pain management. (p. 359)

Cohen (1993) further identifies factors that need consideration in the planning of postoperative pain management (Table 6.1). These factors interlink and need individual consideration to ensure that pain relief and safety are optimized. The type of analgesia management plan and the nursing-based interventions will be governed by the above factors and will indicate the most/least appropriate course of action. The type and site of surgery and the severity of pain expected may indicate the type of analgesia use (opioid or non-opioid) as well as the route of administration (oral, intravenous, patient-controlled analgesia (PCA), topical, regional and so on). The child who has had day surgery will obviously be limited to the milder analgesics or those with a short half-life. Drugs which are commonly used in post-operative analgesic regimes include morphine, papaveretum, pethidine, codeine

Table 6.1 Basic considerations during the development of a postoperative analgesic plan (Cohen, 1993)

Type and site of surgery planned
Severity of pain expected
Predicted recovery course
Abilities of the patient
Patient and family needs and desires
Associated medical and psychological issues
Experience of health care team
Technical aspects of intervention
Environment

phosphate and paracetamol. Additionally drugs such as bupivicaine – a long-lasting local anaesthetic – can successfully be used in local infiltration of the wound before closure. A caudal block can also be used in the management of postoperative pain and can be used in operations such as orchidopexy and herniotomy (Wark, 1991). Other blocks can also provide regional relief of pain postoperatively and children tend to tolerate these well, provided preoperative preparation has been adequate. The child's individual abilities and needs must be assessed in respect to their needs for pain management and the most appropriate choice made. Children who have had a bad experience previously may need a significantly higher input from nursing staff and parents. These children may be over-sensitized (Melamed *et al.*, 1983). Often the child's associated medical problems may create some initial difficulty in choosing the right management approach. This should be considered before surgery so that the child will not suffer whilst a decision is being made. Medical problems such as poor renal function, respiratory instability and cardiovascular instability pose problems which are not insurmountable. The hospital environment is often very worrying to children and can add to their anxiety levels, as can the use of unfamiliar machinery, words and a lack of the reassuring presence of the child's parents and/or the nurse. The pain management programme is only as dynamic, flexible and varied as the resources and skills of the multidisciplinary team using them. Knowledge and competence are required to ensure that the most appropriate method of ensuring pain management is utilized safely and effectively (Cohen, 1993).

The concept of a perioperative treatment ladder is discussed by Cohen (1993), who sees effective management of pain starting before the operation and continuing until the child is pain free and recovered from the procedure (Table 6.2).

Postoperative pain assessment plays a vital role in pain management and appropriate assessment tools are crucial if the nurse is to assess the effectiveness of both pharmacological and non-pharmacological approaches. Arandine *et al.* (1988) found that children as young as 3 years old were able to rate levels of their postoperative pain both before and after analgesia, and

Table 6.2 Therapeutic treatment ladder in perioperative period (Cohen, 1993)

Epoch	Neural action	Interventions
Preoperative	Prevent peripheral and central sensitization	Psychological Opioids NSAIDS
Intraoperative	Decrease/minimize nociceptive impulses	Opioids Local anaesthesia NSAIDs
Postoperative	Minimize nociceptive impulses	Opioids Local anaesthesia NSAIDs Physical Psychological

all the children in the study reported experiencing postoperative pain. Not all children reported that the analgesics used were effective and this indicates the need for frequent reassessment of pain management.

The range of possible interventions is wide and includes the use of PCA using opioids, opioids via intravenous bolus or infusion, NSAIDs, regional blocks, the use of a combination of opioids and non-opioids and non-pharmacological means such as touch, distraction and imagery, and above all the reassuring presence of the nurse and the child's family.

PROCEDURAL PAIN IN CHILDREN

You'll still be taking blood out of me when I'm dead.

(Jonathan, aged 7 years, experiencing
pain from a shingles-type rash)

I have needles lots of time and I just feel a bit shaky, a bit wobbly but I don't tell mum else she gets shaky too . . . sometimes I get dead shaky inside.

(Rachel, aged 9 years)

Procedural pain is a real concern to children and therefore it should be a major concern to nurses caring for children. Although it may be clear to the professionals caring for the child that blood needs to be taken, an intravenous infusion cannula needs to be sited, bone marrow needs to be aspirated, cerebrospinal fluid needs to be obtained and intramuscular injections need to be given, it is rarely obvious to the bewildered child who is in a strange environment in which they are unable to control much, if anything of their destiny. Added to this their parents may also be worried, frightened and unable to protect them from the harm that they see is being inflicted on their child.

Although many invasive and potentially painful procedures may be an inevitable part of a hospital admission the nurse must attempt to limit the number of distressing and painful procedures the child is exposed to and provide adequate preparation and comfort for those that the child must have. Indeed in a recent study by Southall *et al.* (1993) of 55 children (aged 1 month to 12.5 years) in an intensive care unit 181 invasive procedures were recorded with a median duration of 5 minutes. Of these 181 procedures 50 had been performed without any additional analgesia or sedation and 36 of the children had either grimaced or cried. In 89 of the procedures carried out children were recorded as having an adverse response. The numbers of procedures performed on children varied largely depending on the length of stay. One child had a total of 159 procedures performed during an admission to the unit lasting 265 days. One of the findings of the study was that a further 318 procedures had been performed (according to the children's case notes) but had not been recorded. Part of the nurse's role should involve insisting that appropriate analgesics or local anaesthetics are used as an integral part of the procedure during invasive procedures wherever possible (Eland, 1988). This may result in a level of unpopularity with some medical staff but protecting the child is more important. Additionally all painful procedures should be documented in the child's care plan, as should their responses and the pain management strategy. A study by Lander *et al.* (1992) on the influence of technical factors on children's perception of pain showed that technique did not affect the child's perception but that age and anxiety were the two variables that predicted venepuncture pain.

Studies have demonstrated how many children become extremely apprehensive and distressed prior to procedures and that this can intensify the pain experience (Jay *et al.*, 1983; McGrath and deVeber, 1986; Broome *et al.*, 1990). Increasingly the issue of procedural pain is being researched in an attempt to allow effective management to be offered to the child prior to the procedure. Information, preparation and development of coping strategies appear to be the key elements in reducing the pain and distress associated with procedural pain. In improving the child's compliance with a coping technique the nurse must be prepared, and skilled enough, to choose the most appropriate technique for an individual child and their family. Information giving is fundamental to preparing any child and the skill is in giving the information in an appropriate way that the child understands and getting the timing right so that the child does not get anxious about both the information and the procedure. Very young children have little concept of time and they live very much in the present; therefore they should receive their preparation only a short time before otherwise they can become distressed about the information and the prospect of the procedure. Older children tend to prefer to be given longer to internalize the information and prepare themselves. Again it is important that the child's own individual preferences are considered and children should be asked when they want to be told about having another injection or having their dressing changed again and so on.

Information giving should be comprehensive but does not need to be exhaustive. The child will need to have information about what will happen, how long it will take, why it needs to be done, what it will feel like, where it will be done, who will be involved and so on (Anderson and Masur, 1977; Patterson and Lewis Ware, 1988). Månsson *et al.* (1993) studied the effects of preparation programmes on children's reactions to and reports of pain in relation to lumbar puncture for chemotherapy and found that the children who were given the most information had 'sustained reductions in their perceptions of pain'. It is very important to ensure that the child receives not only the preparatory information about what is about to happen but also, if not more importantly, information about how to cope with it. Information alone is not and never will be the sole answer – coping strategies are a crucial part of the preparatory package. Harrison (1991) reports the successful use of a picture book in helping prepare, relax and reduce pain associated with children requiring venous blood sampling. Jay *et al.* (1987) and Zelter and LeBaron (1986) have shown that non-pharmacological approaches such as relaxation, distraction, hypnosis and imagery can be helpful in reducing the pain experienced during painful procedures.

The use of positive reinforcement is often a means of helping the child through the prospect of and the actual experience of the procedure. Children often respond well to the use of bravery certificates, badges and gold stars on a chart at the bottom of their bed. Children can become involved in the prospect of adding stars to their chart, colouring in their certificate during the procedure, and this can act as an element in the use of distraction. Some children become inordinately proud (with good reason) of their collection of bravery certificates that they collect during a hospital admission or whilst cared for at home. It also reminds the nursing and medical staff of the number of procedures that the child has been subjected to. The nurses and the rest of the team should always praise the child and recognize their achievement. Bravery should not be measured against the traditional (and perhaps idiotic) stiff upper lip but in terms of the child's attempts to 'hold still', and use the techniques taught to them (Williams, 1987). Certificates can be individualized for the child and the procedure. It only takes a little care and imagination to provide a suitable certificate for a child. Often the certificates have either current cartoon heroes or the hospital mascot (usually a sad looking teddy or rabbit). Sometimes parents and the child's siblings design special certificates for their child and this makes them extra special and important to the child. Children often compare their certificates and it is not unheard of to witness children swapping certificates as they do with other things:

I have got loads of bravery certificates – I've even got some when I wasn't brave – but they [nurses] still gave them to me and that made me feel OK . . . because mostly I wanted to be brave . . . but it's hard sometimes.

(Julie, aged 10 years)

Some children may benefit from the use of sedation prior to unpleasant, painful procedures. It should be remembered, however, that the sedation will not necessarily have any analgesic effects and that the use of sedation does not magically absolve the nurse from a responsibility to prepare the child. Preparation in this situation will involve preparing the child for the sedation and how it will affect them.

The use of EMLA cream has a major role in preparing children and in reducing the pain associated with some invasive procedures. Clarke and Radford (1986) demonstrated the effect of EMLA in alleviating the pain associated with repeated venepuncture in children with leukaemia. Entonox is also useful in terms of helping children cope with painful procedures – it has been successfully used in the management of burns dressings.

Needles hurt but not that much 'cos I have EMLA on – it's a bit smelly but I like it because the needles are better – I like helping the nurse put it on – it's good to do that.

(James, aged 8 years)

For the child the painful procedure does not stop as soon as the needle is out or the dressing is back on again – they need time to recover and the nurse should take time to be with the child after the procedure rather than simply rush off. Children appreciate praise and will often like to tell the nurse how 'good' they were and how they 'were the bravest ever'. This time after the procedure can be a good experience for the nurse, who is able to recharge caring batteries after having been involved in some part of the pain infliction process.

Children can be prepared for painful procedures – it takes time, care and imagination on the nurse's part and the rewards are obvious when the child copes better, is less frightened, recovers more quickly and does not completely dread the daily bloods or tests.

CHRONIC PAIN IN CHILDREN

Varni and Walco (1988) state that paediatric chronic pain is typically characterized by:

the absence of an anxious component, with a constellation of reactive features such as compensatory posturing, lack of developmentally appropriate behaviors, depressed mood, and inactivity or restriction in the normal activities of daily living. These chronic pain behaviors

may eventually be maintained independently of the original nociceptive impulses (pain sensations) and tissue damage, being reinforced
by socioenvironmental influences. (p. 146)

In consideration of a definition as gloomy as that given above, obviously the
nurse has a central role in minimizing the widespread harm that chronic pain
can cause. Chronic pain hurts more than just physically – it has the capacity
to hurt everything in the child's life. For children experiencing chronic pain
such as the recurrent acute type of the vaso-occlusive crises of sickle cell
disease, the chronic benign pain experienced in rheumatoid arthritis and the
chronic acute pain experienced by some children with terminal cancer,
complete pain relief may not be a practical or realistic goal. Newburger and
Sallan (1981) propose that in some cases there needs to be a balance between
the child's functional ability and a reduction in the pain experience. However,
the aim must surely be to reduce the pain to the lowest achievable level that
still maintains a good quality of life.

One of the major problems and the fundamental difference between acute
and chronic pain for the child and their family is the impact that it has on
everyone's lives – sometimes on many aspects of their lives. Beales (1986)
suggests that chronic pain may be a cause for 'profound misery'. Chronic
pain can disturb the child's emotional, physical and social development (Hodges
et al., 1985; Webster, 1993). Chronic pain management must above all have
the potential handicapping and disabling features of the effects of pain as a
prime concern. The child's understanding of the meaning and relevance of
their pain and their expectations in regard to relief of that pain are important
aspects of the child's experience of pain and subsequent management (Beales
et al., 1983). As with shorter-duration acute pain, a child's understanding
can impact in a major way on their whole experience; a lack of understanding tends to exacerbate the experience and children are less able to cope
with and control their pain (McGrath,1990).

Since chronic pain is often associated with an illness such as juvenile
rheumatoid arthritis, sickle cell disease, haemophilia and so on, the child
and their family not only have to cope with the pain which is part of the
underlying disease itself but also contend with the pain associated with the
investigations required in the management of the disease process. This can
add immeasurably to the child's pain load and they should be encouraged
to learn coping strategies such as distraction, relaxation, and imagery if they
are to feel able to deal with the situation. Children's emotional ability to
handle the disease will impact on their experience of the associated pain (Beales
et al., 1983).

Spitzer (1993) in a study of how children (aged 6–13 years) with haemophilia
described their experience with pain in relation to understanding their illness
and treatment experience showed that pain was seen to be a major part of
their concerns and seen to be a great threat. Spitzer reports that the children

appeared to try and categorize types of pain into ones which were tolerable and those which were not. The younger children described pain as making them feel 'bad' and 'sad' – the two words being used interchangeably. Importantly this study highlighted a new aspect of how children understand and relate to their pain.

> Pain had two major functions within children's illness experiences: a severity indicator and a communication mode between the child, the family, and the health care team. As such pain had a critical role in (a) helping children with hemophilia assess changes to their health and (b) communicating the changes to their parents or caregivers to assure timely intervention. (Spitzer, 1993, p. 16)

Children who have experienced chronic pain for a prolonged period of time may exhibit pain in a more obvious, expressive way. This can result in a negative effect in terms of the family being tempted to or actively trying to ignore the child's responses as a means of attempting to reduce the frequency or intensity of the behaviour (McCaffery and Beebe, 1989; Mathews *et al.*, 1993). Trying to manage pain by simply reducing the expression of the child's pain does not work – it simply hides the pain problem and does not solve or resolve it. However, McCaffery and Beebe (1989) report that this may often occur as the health care team are held:

> accountable for controlling the patient's *expression* of pain . . . we are asking the patient to suffer in silence, to learn to live with his pain and leave us alone. (p. 2)

Obviously this is inappropriate and unethical since nurses as part of the multidisciplinary team must accept responsibility for managing pain.

Merskey and Spear (1967) suggest that children who experience chronic pain are more likely to experience chronic pain as adults. Families can have a major impact on the way in which children cope with chronic pain – parents who encourage their children to cope with and overcome some of the potentially disabling aspects of pain can help to reduce the impact and intensity of pain (Mathews *et al.*, 1993).

Of course the type of chronic pain will influence the pain management programme but there is definitely a place for the non-pharmacological, therapeutic interventions, as these can provide a means of control over the pain, the symptoms and the disease itself.

Juvenile rheumatoid arthritis

Juvenile rheumatoid arthritis (JRA) is a syndrome with peak periods of onset between 18 months to 5 years and 8½–12 years (Brunner and Suddarth, 1991). It is one of the most frequently occurring chronic illnesses presenting in childhood and a major cause of disability (Cassidy, 1991). Characteristic symptoms include swollen joints that are tender, painful and hot, accompanied by limited movement (Ludwig and Beam, 1992). Three subtypes of disease onset are recognized: systemic onset, polyarticular onset and pauciarticular onset. Systemic onset accounts for about 20% of the total population of JRA and is characterized by abrupt fever and rash. Polyarticular JRA is characterized by arthritis in five or more joints and accounts for about 40–50% of children with JRA. Pauciarticular JRA is characterized by four or fewer joints being affected and accounts for the remaining 40–50% of children with JRA (Cassidy, 1991; Page, 1991; Walco and Oberlander, 1993). The pain experienced by children with JRA varies from a dull ache through to a dull, constant pain to intense pain (Ross and Ross, 1988). Morning stiffness, night pain and 'gelling' after inactivity are characteristic of JRA. Beales et al. (1983) provide information about the child's perception of the disease. In this study children (aged 6–17 years) with JRA were interviewed about their joint sensations and the meaning that they felt that these sensations had. The younger children in the study (6–11 years) did not appear to link the joint sensations with the underlying disorder, but the older children were able to make this link. Additionally the younger children reported less pain severity than the older children. Adolescents may become very distressed at the 'imagined implications' of the pain and of the effect that it is having on them socially and emotionally (Beales, 1986). This perhaps provides a clue that children need different types of support from nursing staff. The older children need psychological support in dealing with the pain that they associate with a potentially disabling disease, whilst the younger children may need to be warned not to over-exert 'at-risk' joints.

The small amount of research focused on the needs of JRA children and their pain shows that the pain is clearly associated with the severity of the disease, the way in which the family cope, the child's physical limitations and their psychological adjustment.

A study by Walco et al. (1990) demonstrated that children with JRA had pain thresholds significantly lower than healthy children in the study, which may indicate that they have been sensitized by their previous experiences of pain. Varni and Walco (1988) advocate the use of a multidimensional approach to assessment of children with JRA to allow comprehensive management to occur so that 'potentially modifiable psychological and socio-environmental factors' (p. 153) can be identified. The Varni–Thompson Pediatric Pain Questionnaire (PPQ) allows the child's pain to be comprehensively assessed and Page (1991) suggests that the PPQ is a:

> desirable inventory for establishing a data base for individualising the care of a child diagnosed with JRA. (p. 21)

Intervention strategies for JRA are not fully developed and it is the symptoms that tend to be treated. Treatment is supportive and drug therapy aims to reduce inflammation and provide analgesia (Brunner and Suddarth,

1991). Pharmacological management is based initially on NSAIDs such as aspirin which act to suppress pain and inflammation. Due to the reported association between aspirin and Reye's syndrome Cassidy (1991) reports that salicylates are discontinued for about 14 days during outbreaks of varicella and influenza and vaccination against influenza is recommended as a precautionary measure. Page (1991) reports that aspirin is more frequently associated with gastrointestinal side-effects and elevated liver enzymes, and other NSAIDs may need to be trialled. Other drug therapies include the use of gold salts, corticosteroid drugs and immunosuppressive drugs. Non-pharmacological methods are useful in allowing the child to take control, and simple measures such as keeping the joints warm at night, warm baths and gentle exercises have been reported to reduce morning stiffness (Page-Goertz, 1989). Varni and Walco (1988) suggest that the use of guided imagery, progressive muscle relaxation and meditative breathing have the potential to be a valuable part of pain management in JRA children. Therapies such as massage and aromatherapy can be useful in relaxing tense skeletal muscles and by the judicious use of anti-inflammatory and diuretic oils can help to calm and relieve swollen and painful joints (Day, 1995). Walco and Oberlander (1993) report that self-regulatory techniques have led to a reduction in pain intensity and an improvement in adaptive functioning with children with JRA.

Sickle cell pain

Sickle cell pain falls into the category of chronic pain labelled recurrent acute and the vaso-occlusive crises can result in acute, intensely painful experiences that can last from hours to days. Repeated chronic pain can have a major impact on the child's normal activities, including school attendance, school progress, and sleep quality and quantity (Shapiro et al., 1970). Sickle cell disease is an inherited disorder which mostly affects ethnic groups from areas in which malaria is endemic, such as Africa, India and the Mediterranean. The approach to managing sickle cell pain is through hydration and analgesia. Pain is the most frequent symptom of sickle cell disease (Morrison and Vedro, 1989). The painful crisis can be classified as producing either mild, moderate or severe episodes. The severe episodes produce intense, agonizing pain that needs effective and urgent attention. Children with sickle cell disease will often face the prospect of repeated attacks of pain with their crises and it is essential that each and every crisis is managed effectively and with care so that the child's anxiety levels are not increased unnecessarily. Shapiro et al. (1990) suggest that children experiencing repeated vaso-occlusive crisis pain may additionally experience 'significant depression, psychosocial dysfunction, and inability to pursue an independent lifestyle (p. 314). One problem that children face in respect to sickle cell pain is a degree of ignorance on the part of many professionals who have limited knowledge and experience of caring for such children. The Sickle Cell and Thalassaemia Association of Counsellors (STAC) recognizes that a major need is to improve education and understanding of sickle cell and some of the biased attitudes held about sickle cell sufferers. Shankleman and May (1993) in a preface to the proceedings of a conference on sickle cell pain highlight some of the difficulties that patients in severe pain may experience: they may be labelled as 'junkies' or 'addicts'; seen to display drug-seeking behaviour; and are at risk of being treated with contempt and resentment. Some of these attitudes may originate in the fact that most sickle cell sufferers are black and the majority of health professionals are white. Ethnic, cultural and social differences may result in a degree of misinterpretation of the experience by professionals (Shapiro, 1993). Schechter *et al*. (1988) report that sickle cell pain is inadequately treated due to an amalgam of issues (Fig. 6.1).

In a study by Gill *et al*. (1991) the children in the study were seen to be either high copers or low copers. The high copers were more active and required less frequent health care, whilst the children who appeared to be more passive needed more input from health care professionals and were more negative in their thinking.

Sickle cell crises vary from child to child and not every child will experience intense pain. However, painful crises need to be managed with opioid analgesia and often large doses are required to provide effective management. Sartori *et al*. (1990) report successful use of continuous infusion of papavertum for the severe sickling crisis of 24 children on 45 occasions (1.7–14.3 years). The dose of papaveretum was titrated against effect and based on assessment

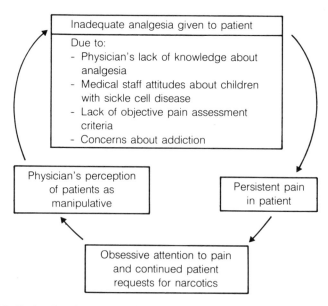

Figure 6.1 Cycle of undertreatment (Schechter *et al*., 1988).

using a faces scale in some of the children. The researchers noted a consistent increase of dosage per kilogram with age which may have been related to either an increase in severity with age or perhaps an improvement in their ability to communicate pain. Morrison and Vedro (1989) recommend the use of continuous infusion of morphine and meperidine (pethidine) although subsequent research has provided evidence that meperidine is not suitable due to the fact that sickle cell patients are at risk from normeperidine-induced seizures (normeperidine is a metabolite of meperidine which can induce seizures and hallucinations (Tong *et al.*, 1980). Meperidine was among the drugs used in a survey by Pegelow (1992). Shapiro (1993) recommends that the use of oral opioids should be considered whenever possible as they may take the 'drama out of the crisis' and reduce the psychological impact that repeated hospital admission with intravenous therapy may cause.

PCA may have a place to play in the management of crises, especially as the child is legitimately in control of the amount of analgesia required – pain management is likely to be optimal and side-effects lower (Harmar, 1993; Holbrook, 1990; Schechter *et al.*, 1988). Schechter *et al.* report PCA to be a 'theoretically sound and technically feasible' treatment option.

The role of nursing intervention and non-pharmacological approaches is again a vital one in the management of children with sickle cell. The children and their family need to be involved in their care and management, and trust is a vital part of this relationship. Burghardt-Fitzgerald (1989) reports the use of pain behaviour contracts as a means of helping adolescents manage their pain, improve compliance with their care and reduce any maladaptive or inappropriate behaviour. The contract is develped in negotiation with the child and includes therapies and activities based on different levels that correspond to pain experienced. Shapiro *et al.* (1990) report the viability of using a daily diary as a means of collecting information about children experiencing vaso-occlusive crisis. The importance of this method of gathering information is that it reflects the child's perception of the impact that the pain has on them and their life. The authors additionally propose that subsequent decisions about pain management strategies can be based on 'real-time' information. Children with sickle cell disease have time between periods of pain to be prepared for any subsequent periods of pain. This means that the child should be given information about how their pain will be managed, what they can do to help themselves, learn how to use self-hypnosis, imagery and so on, and how to use the pain assessment tool (Pegelow, 1992). If the child has a good level of preparation it is likely that the pain experience will be less frightening and the pain experienced less intense.

NEONATAL PAIN

Until recently, it was generally accepted within the medical and nursing profession that the neonate was incapable of experiencing pain. This assumption became a persistent and pervasive myth that dominated the understanding (or perhaps more correctly misunderstanding) and attitudes towards neonatal pain. Purcell-Jones *et al.* (1988) suggests the fact that pain has been overlooked does not necessarily demonstrate a lack of concern but rather it shows that the assumptions on which the thinking was based was outdated and incorrect. That this myth developed is somewhat surprising, especially when the crucial need for pain as a protection and warning system is otherwise generally accepted. Indeed Grunau and Craig (1987) highlight this need when they comment:

> In bioevolutionary terms, for species survival neonatal sensitivity to pain and a highly developed means of communicating pain to the caretaker appears essential and fundamental. (p. 407)

Early research proposed that the neonate was incapable of experiencing pain due to immaturity and inactivity of the neonate's cerebral cortex, lack of emotional development and undeveloped pain pathways (Angulo and Gonzales, 1929; Langworthy, 1933; McGraw, 1941). However, more recent studies refute this; Volpe (1981) demonstrated that complete myelination of the neurones was not a necessary prerequisite for pain to be experienced. Anand and Hickey (1987) stated that:

> newborns do have the anatomical and functional components required for the perception of painful stimulus. (p. 1323)

The neurophysiological basis for pain reception and relay is present well before birth. The fetal cortex starts to develop at eight weeks gestation and by the 20th week of gestation the cortex has its full complement of approximately 10^9 neurones (Anand and Hickey, 1987). Eland and Anderson (1977) report that between the 20th and 24th week of gestation the connection is made between the cerebral cortex and the thalamus and that synaptogenesis develops. Beyer and Wells (1989) suggest that due to the neonate's size the intraneuronal distance is comparatively much shorter than that of an adult and that this acts as a compensation for the fact that myelination of the nerves is incomplete. Anand and Carr (1989) and Anand and Hickey (1987) report that the fetus's cortex is functionally mature well before birth, and Booker (1987) suggests that it may be possible for neonates to experience pain at the cortical level. Fitzgerald *et al.* (1989) report that the preterm neonate has a lower threshold to potentially noxious stimuli compared with the full-term neonate. Work by Fitzgerald (1985) demonstrates that increased sensitization occurs following stimulation which may be due to a lack of inhibitory control in the immature spinal cord. Torres and Anderson (1985) have shown evoked cortical activity in response to auditory, olfactory and tactile stimuli in preterm babies.

With the increase in evidence supporting the neurophysiological basis for pain and the developing evidence drawn from studies demonstrating the physiological and behavioural responses evoked by painful stimuli such as heel stick and circumcision and other postoperative pain, attitudes to pain management are having to change (Cote *et al.*, 1991; Craig *et al.*, 1993; Grunau and Craig, 1987; Johnston *et al.*, 1993; McIntosh *et al.*, 1993; McLaughlin *et al.*, 1993; Owens and Todt, 1984; Williamson and Williamson, 1983).

It is no longer possible for professionals to neglect this issue – the time for acting upon the evidence is now (Carter, 1990). Owens (1984) summed up some of the major factors contributing to the mismanagement of neonatal pain when he stated:

> For years, researchers and clinicians have made assumptions about whether infants experience pain based on casual observations or theoretical indifference. (p. 213)

As a result of this casual and indifferent approach analgesia and anaesthesia have been actively withheld.

Professional attitudes at the clinical level are changing. Booker (1987) in a survey of anaesthetists found that 40% of the respondents never provided postoperative analgesia of any kind to neonates during or after major surgery. In 1987 the American Academy of Pediatrics issued a statement on the appropriate use of neonatal anaesthesia which aims to give neonates the same consideration/rights as older patients in respect to anaesthesia. McLaughlin *et al.* (1993) surveyed 352 neonatal and perinatal specialists in America about attitudes and practices to infant pain and pain management in spontaneously breathing infants. Most respondents indicated that even the most premature infants (less than 28 weeks gestation) are able to perceive pain and most advocated anaesthesia during the intraoperative period. Those who indicated that neonates do not feel less pain than adults saw more signs of pain and used more medication postoperatively. The converse was also true with those who believed that the infant is less sensitive, giving less. There was a lack of consensus about the 'fact' that physiological stress can be more dangerous than analgesia – respondents simply acknowledged that they did not know.

Neonatal pain research has centred on two procedures: heel stab and circumcision. These two procedures are used as they give rise to bright, easily localized cutaneous pain. Initially research centred on healthy term neonates' response to pain although more work is now in progress related to the preterm neonates' responses (Craig *et al.*, 1993; Johnston *et al.*, 1993). Responses noted have been classified under behavioural and physiological headings. The physiological responses include heart rate, blood pressure, respiratory rate, palmar sweating, respiratory rate, oxygenation and metabolic and endocrine changes (Anand *et al.*, 1985; Beaver, 1987; Brown, 1987; Gunnar *et al.*, 1981; Owens and Todt, 1984; Williamson and Williamson, 1988). The behavioural responses include facial expression, crying and body movement (Cote *et al.*, 1991; Franck, 1985; Grunau and Craig, 1987; Grunau *et al.*,

1990; Levine and Gordon, 1982; Izard, 1971; Porter, 1989; Wolff, 1969, 1974). Behavioural responses are generally more difficult to record, measure and document when compared with the 'harder' physiological data. However, behavioural responses are probably the most valuable piece of communication that is occurring. Some of the early research focused on healthy term infants, which was important in providing information on their responses, but perhaps what is of more clinical interest is the response of the sick, vulnerable and preterm infants who populate the neonatal intensive care units. The infants have minimal reserves of strength and their pain responses may have potentially catastrophic consequences. However, despite the overwhelming evidence there is still not an established neonatal pain assessment tool and nearly all assessment is made subjectively and perhaps intuitively – even though this subjective judgement is based somewhat loosely on behavioural and physiological responses. Interestingly, a study by Elander et al. (1991) suggests that parents have the same level of awareness of their infant's pain as the nurses caring for the infant. In this respect the parents must be seen as a valuable resource in terms of the assessment of pain and this again is an example of the opportunities of being able to work in partnership with the parents in a very real and valuable way.

Treatment and management of neonatal pain is complex and requires a multidimensional approach. Skilled therapeutic nursing care will always be required to complement drug regimes and the other therapies. The use of a range of aids to ensure that the baby is comfortable needs to be considered, including bean bags, soft rolls, good positioning to reduce pressure and traction on wounds, maintenance of an atraumatic environment that protects the baby from unnecessary noise, limiting the volume of handling and disturbance, providing the baby with a 'nest' around them to allow them to be in touch with the limits of their environment and encouraging rest and sleep. All these measures will provide a basic and vital level of nursing care and pain management. The stress and distress that are associated with pain are likely to be reduced. All procedures should be grouped and procedures should be reduced to a therapeutic minimum (Vandenberg and Franck, 1990). Routine procedures, such as heel stab, can be made less traumatic and thus not add to the overall pain load by using the best technique. McIntosh et al. (1993) in a study of heel stab in 35 preterm babies (26–34 weeks gestation) aged 5–35 days old found that EMLA cream did not help as it appeared to create vaso-constriction and increased squeezing was required, and comforting measures were helpful. However, the most successful way of decreasing the distress/pain response was to use a glucolet rather than a lance. Myron and Maguire (1991) propose that infants be comforted by a soothing voice, a pacifier and close boundaries after a heel stab. Care, however, does need to be taken when considering soothing a baby by talking, as Beaver (1987) showed that nurses touching and talking to the baby after painful procedures could result in a a further drop in tcPO$_2$ levels. Work by Marchette *et al.* (1991) studied the use of classical music, intrauterine sounds, pacifier, music and pacifier, and intrauterine sounds and pacifier on 121 neonates undergoing unanaesthetized circumcision. None of the above interventions greatly reduced the pain as determined by physiological variables, although sucking did appear to decrease crying in the group that had both the pacifier and the intrauterine sounds. Gunnar *et al.* (1984) report on the effects of a pacifier on the adrenocortical and behavioural responses to circumcision in 18 healthy term infants (2–5 days old). The group was divided into a control group (no pacifier) and the pacifier group. There were no significant differences reported in the adreno-cortical responses although the pacifier group cried for 35% less time than the control group.

Neonates obviously prove problematic in respect to the management of their pain; however, that in itself is insufficient reason not to attempt effective pain relief. Elander *et al.* (1991) report that in a study of postoperative pain management in infants aged 0–12 months seven out of the nine infants (2.5–5.5 kg weight) received no pain relief despite obvious observable changes to both behaviour and physiological parameters. This study highlights deficits in knowledge, persisting misconceptions about pain management and, perhaps more worryingly, a strange attitude. Nurses are quoted as saying:

> The parents are very brave and keep telling us we can postpone pain relief to the infant.

> We do not follow a schedule; if we did, we might give pain relief to an infant who did not need it.

Pharmacological methods of pain relief in the neonate are now being used more frequently although special attention must be made to consideration of the volume and rate that the drug needs to be given at, fluid restrictions, the required dilution of the drug, and the neonate's immature kidneys and liver. The choice of analgesia depends on the infant's diagnosis, site of pain, general condition, nature and expected duration of the pain, and the resources available for the administration of the drug and the support available for the neonate should respiratory depression or other side-effects occur. Very sick neonates requiring opioids, such as morphine and fentanyl, for pain management characteristically show delayed excretion of the drug and the elimination half-life is prolonged, which may result in the drugs accumulating (Goldman and Lloyd-Thomas, 1991). The need for resources for resuscitation are highlighted as a key issue by Purcell-Jones *et al.* (1987).

Purcell-Jones *et al.* (1987) reported a retrospective study of 933 cases of use of opioids in neonates. This study showed an increase in the use of opioids in neonates over the five-year period (1980–1984) from 9.7% to 27.2% of admitted cases. Four babies in the study failed to wean from controlled ventilation, which was seen to be a result of opioid-induced respiratory depression. Seven of the 51 spontaneously breathing infants developed respiratory failure or apnoea, which was felt to be induced by the opioids. Codeine phosphate (intramuscularly) was the most commonly used opioid in the spontaneously breathing group and morphine sulphate in the ventilated group. Koren *et al.* (1985) suggest that continuous morphine infusion can be safe and effective provided the dose is safe – the neonate's reduced plasma binding capacity means that the required dose is only small. Preterm neonates also have delayed terminal elimination half-lives and delayed clearance of morphine compared to older neonates (Franck and Gregory, 1993). Due to the immaturity of the blood–brain barrier there is an increased degree of permeability that results in increased concentrations of endogenous opioids in the cerebrospinal fluid and in the blood (Orlowski, 1986).

Fentanyl has been reported as being effective and causing few problems (Anand *et al.*, 1987) although respiratory complications have been reported (Hertzke *et al.*, 1984). The use of local anaesthetic is an important issue to consider. Williamson and Williamson (1983) found firm evidence of the effectiveness of lidocaine as a local anaesthetic and suggest that its use could be widened to allow procedures such as the insertion of chest drains to be performed with minimal pain. Goldman and Lloyd-Thomas (1991) report that bupivicaine plain has a good safety record with neonates. They also acknowledge that whilst a range of blocks and wound infiltration can be used for neonates for postoperative pain management they are still rarely used for one of the most common neonatal operations – circumcision. This seems particularly unfortunate since much of the data that has been produced to convince professionals that neonates do experience pain and its repercussions have come from this group. Yaster (1987) is categorical in his belief that:

> Local infiltration of the skin is so safe that there is little, if any, reason ever to perform a cutdown for vascular access without its use. (p. 395)

Berry and Gregory (1987) propose that apart from the moribund infant very small, sick, preterm infants can be anaesthetized safely. However, preterm neonates are clearly at more risk with anaesthesia than their term counterparts. They tend to become more stressed by anaesthesia and are particularly sensitive to the cardiodepressant and ventilatory depressant effects of anaesthesia (Diaz, 1991). However, many of the problems that are posed by the preterm neonate can be overcome provided the anaesthetist is a specialist. Barrier *et al.* (1989) showed the effectiveness of minor postoperative analgesia (fentanyl versus placebo) by looking at a variety of factors.

Neonates are a special case but they must be considered to be prime candidates for inclusion in pain management strategies. Small as they are, they too have a right to pain relief. Fitzgerald (1991) warns that neonatal pain must be taken seriously owing to the vulnerability of their developing nervous systems and the potential for the noxious stimuli they are exposed to having a diffuse and possible profound effect.

ONCOLOGY PAIN

> When I'm sick I get pain all the way down my side and I retch for ages and that's sore and awful ... I think people [nurses] think that it [pain] will just go away but it doesn't it still hurts even when I've stopped being sick and it hurts my throat and makes it burn ... my head hurt when my hair was falling out – it hurt all over and I didn't know what to do but I just told my mum and she said I'd be OK ... Sometimes I just hurt a little bit in lots of places and that's bad because they make each other worse but if I told them [nurses] they'd just think I was being silly and moaning 'cos they couldn't do much about it – but it helps if they stay with me and talk – yes that helps.
>
>   (Jennifer, aged 12 years receiving chemotherapy)

Children with cancer may well experience pain from a multiplicity of sources: the pain associated with the cancer/tumour itself; the pain associated with the investigations and the management of the disease process; and the pain associated with dealing with diagnosis and prognosis. Children with cancer may experience pain from compression of nerves, infiltration of integument or tissues, bone destruction, obstructed viscus, ischaemia, inflammation, infection and necrosis (Hockenberry and Coody, 1986). The pain experienced from these underlying pathologies is often intense and can be very frightening for the child. Children may blame themselves for 'getting cancer' and this makes the issue of dealing with the pain more complicated (McGrath and Unruh, 1987). It is obvious therefore that a multidimensional approach to the care of the child is vital and that the child's emotional, social and spiritual needs are met along with their physical needs. The family are a vital component in the care of the child and they will need significant amounts of support to help them adjust to their child's diagnosis and what is going to be expected of them. Cornalgia et al. (1984) report that 57% of children with cancer in the study experienced moderate to severe pain during their treatment. McGrath and Unruh (1987) report that pain is problematic for children with cancer. Miser et al. (1987a) found that in 72 out of 92 newly diagnosed patients pain was the presenting symptom. Miser et al. (1987b) reported that pain was experienced by 25% of outpatients and 50% of hospitalized children and that it was generally treatment-associated pain. However, 33% of the children in this study experienced tumour-related pain. Sutters and Miaskowski (1992) propose that chronic persistent pain (intractable pain lasting longer than six months) is perhaps less common in children than in adults with cancer since 'children with unresponsive or refractory malignancies usually experience a rapid demise' (p. 466). However, further research may well uncover a different picture of the pain associated with childhood malignancy.

Many of the studies associated with pain and children with cancer have concentrated on procedural pain (Broome *et al.*, 1990; Mansson *et al.*, 1993), which is important but the other sources of pain must not be overlooked in terms of both management and research. Children with cancer pains need to have these pains accurately assessed and time must be taken in the assessment process to allow the child to talk about their pain in a free and unstructured way. A comprehensive pain assessment tool that does not simply focus on the intensity of the pain should be utilized so that the quality, nature, intensity, meaning, limitations and fears related to the pain can be documented, evaluated and acted upon. This is important since the pain which may appear to be the main problem from the nurse's perspective may not be the most difficult one to cope with for the child. Pain or the fear of intractable pain may be a major worry for the child and their family and this must be accepted by the nurse and reassurance given that pain management will be seen to be a priority within the overall package of care (Goldman *et al.*, 1990). Hockenberry and Coody (1986) propose that the nurse must discuss realistic pain relief goals with the child and their family and that these

Table 6.3 Analgesic interventions for children with cancer pain (from Miser, 1993)

Anticancer treatment[a]
Radiotherapy
Chemotherapy
Biological therapy
Surgery
Analgesic drugs[b]
Non-invasive techniques
Transcutaneous nerve stimulation
Physical therapy
Hypnosis
Relaxation
Biofeedback
Neurosurgical interventions
Regional nerve blocks
Inhalational anaesthetic agents
Supportive counselling

[a] Of primary importance.

[b] Administered alone or in conjunction with other interventions.

goals must be made known to all members of the multidisciplinary team. Miser (1993) identified the range of interventions possible in the management of oncology pain (Table 6.3). However, despite the range of treatments Miser et al. (1987a) found that in the study of children with cancer 29% of those who reported moderate to severe pain were not prescribed analgesics and the remaining 71% had ineffective oral medication. This is obviously an impossible situation for the child and one which should not be allowed to happen. Rational pain management is something which should be available to all children.

The concept of the analgesic ladder is important in managing cancer pain as it allows the progression of analgesics to occur from mild through moderate to strong. The chosen drugs should be given at regular intervals throughout the day so that the child receives continuous analgesia cover rather than experiencing pain associated with a 'trough' in the medication levels. A child who is secure in the knowledge that their pain is being managed is much more likely to be able to carry on the normal activities of living without worrying about the effects of pain. The best route for analgesic administration for the child with chronic cancer pain is oral as it basically involves very little technology and, best of all for the child, no needles. For the child requiring strong opioid pain management slow-release morphine may be the answer as it is active over a 12-hour period. This means that the child has the opportunity for uninterrupted sleep at night and there is a decreased need for frequent medication (Goldman and Bowman, 1990). The dose can be titrated for effect against the child's pain (Goldman et al., 1993). Morphine can also be administered via a continuous intravenous infusion (Dothage et al., 1986; Miser et al., 1980) and by the subcutaneous route if the oral route is not tolerated. This route has proved successful and the child is not at risk from building up a tolerance to the drug that is associated with the intravenous route.

Children with cancer benefit greatly from learning coping strategies since they can help manage both the pain but also the stress and distress that can accompany pain and the disease process itself. Distraction, hypnosis, massage, aromatherapy and the other non-pharmacologically based nursing interventions have a vital role to play within the management of cancer pain (Hilgard and LeBaron, 1984; Hockenberry, 1988; Olness, 1981). Some studies have already been undertaken to demonstrate the value of these therapies as adjunctive measures in the management of severe pain and some of them will help to reduce symptoms such as nausea and anxiety. Above all they return some level of control to the child and their family over even just one aspect of their illness.

The child who is diagnosed with a malignancy is not condemned to a future of pain and suffering. Pain management is a vital part in maintaining the child's quality of life through treatment to either cure or a pain-free death.

REFERENCES

Alex, M.R. and Ritchie, J.A. (1992) School-aged children's interpretation of their experience with acute surgical pain. *Journal of Pediatric Nursing*, **7**(3): 171–180.

American Academy of Pediatrics (1987) Neonatal anesthesia. *Pediatrics*, **80**: 446.

Anand, K.J.S. and Carr, D.B. (1989) The neuroanatomy, neurophysiology, and neurochemistry of pain, stress, and analgesia in newborns and children. *Pediatric Clinics of North America*, **36**(4): 795–882.

Anand, K.J.S., and Hickey, P.R. (1987) Pain and its effects in the human neonate and fetus. *New England Journal of Medicine* **317**(21): 1321–1327.

Anand, K.J.S., Brown, M.J. and Causon, R.C. (1985) Can the human neonate mount an endocrine/metabolic response to surgery? *Journal of Pediatric Surgery*, January: 41–48.

Anand, K.J.S., Sippell, W.G. and Aynsley-Green, A. (1987) A randomised trial of fentanyl anaesthesia in pre-term neonates undergoing surgery: effects on the stress response. *Lancet*, **i**: 243–248.

Anderson, K. and Masur, F. (1977) Psychological preparation for invasive medical and dental procedures. *Journal of Behavioral Medicine*, **6**: 1–40.

Angulo, Y. and Gonzales, A.W. (1929) Is myelinogeny an absolute index of behavioral capability? *Journal of Comprehensive Neurology*, **48**: 459.

Arandine, C.R., Beyer, J.E. and Tompkins, J.M. (1988) Children's pain perception before and after analgesia: a study of instrument construct validity and related issues. *Journal of Pediatric Nursing*, **3**(1): 11–23.

Beales, J.G. (1986) Cognitive development and the experience of pain. *Nursing*, **11**: 408–410.

Beales, J.G., Keen, J.H. and Holt, P.J. (1983) The child's perception of the disease and the experience of pain in juvenile chronic arthritis. *Journal of Rheumatology*, **10**: 61–65.

Beaver, P.K. (1987) Premature infants' response to touch and pain: can nurses make a difference? *Neonatal Network*, **6**(3): 13–17.

Benham, M. and Murray, F. (1993) Regional anaesthesia for pain relief in children *TECHNIC* **115**: 4–5.

Berry, F.A. and Gregory, G.A. (1987) Do premature infants require anesthesia for surgery? *Anesthesia*, **63**(3): 291–293.

Beyer, J.E. and Wells, N. (1989) The assessment of pain in children. *Pediatric Clinics of North America*, **36**(4), 837–854.

Beyer, J.E., DeGood, D.E., Ashley, L.C. and Russell, G.A. (1983) Patterns of post-operative analgesic use with adults and children following cardiac surgery. *Pain*, **17**: 71–81.

Booker, P.D. (1987) Postoperative analgesia for neonates. *Anaesthesia*, **42**: 343–345.

Broome, M.E., Bates, T.A., Lillis, P.P.Y. and Wilson McGahee, T. (1990) Children's medical fears, coping behaviors, and pain perceptions during a lumbar puncture. *Oncology Nursing Forum*, **17**(3): 361–367.

Brown, L. (1987) Physiological response to cutaneous pain in neonates. *Neonatal Network*, **6**(3): 18–22.

Brunner, L.S. and Suddarth, D.S. (1991) *The Lippincott Manual of Pediatric Nursing*, 3rd edn (adapted for UK by Weller, B.F.). Harper Collins, London.

Burghardt-Fitzgerald, D.C. (1989) Pain–behavior contracts: effective management of the adolescent in sickle-cell crisis. *Journal of Pediatric Nursing*, **4**(5): 320–324.

Burokas, L. (1985) Factors affecting nurses decisions to mediate pediatric patients after surgery. *Heart and Lung*, **14**: 373–378.

Carter, B. (1990) A universal experience. *Paediatric Nursing*, Sept: 8–10.

Carter, M.B. (1989) *The Perception of Pain in the Neonate*. Unpublished thesis, Manchester Metropolitan University, Manchester.

Cassidy, J.T. (1991) Connective tissue diseases and amyloidosis. In: Oski, F.A., DeAngelis, C.D., Feigin, R.D. and Warshaw, R.E. (eds), *Principles and Practice of Pediatrics*. Lippincott, Philadelphia, pp. 226–249.

Cohen, D. (1993) Management of postoperative pain in children. In: Schechter, N.L., Berde, C.B. and Yaster, M. (eds), *Pain in Infants, Children and Adolescents*. Williams & Wilkins, Baltimore, pp. 357–383.

Cornalgia, C., Massimo, L., Haupt, R., Melodie, A., Sizemre, W. and Benedetti, C. (1984) Incidence of pain in children with neoplastic disease. *Pain* (suppl.) 2: S28.

Cote, J.J., Morse, J.M. and James, S.G. (1991) The pain response of the postoperative newborn. *Journal of Advanced Nursing*, **16**: 378–387.

Craig, K.D. Whitfield, M.F., Grunan, R.V.E., Linton, J. and Hadjistravropoulas, H.D. (1993) Pain in the preterm neonate: behavioural and physiological indices. *Pain*, 52: 287–299.

Dalens, B. (1993) Peripheral nerve blockade in the management of postoperative pain in children. In: Schechter, N.L., Berde, C.B. and Yaster, M. (eds), *Pain in Infants, Children, and Adolescents*. Williams & Wilkins, Baltimore, pp. 261–280.

Day, S. (1995) Complementary therapies. In: Carter, B. and Dearmun, A.K. (eds) *Child Health Care Nursing: Concepts, Theory and Practice*. Blackwell Scientific Publications, Oxford. (In press)

Dothage, J.A., Arndt, C. and Miser, A.W. (1986) Use of a continuous intravenous morphine infusion for pain control in an infant with terminal malignancy. *Journal of the Association of Oncology Nursing*, 3(4): 22–24.

Douglas, J. (1993) *Psychology and Nursing Children*. Macmillan, Basingstoke.

Eiser, C. and Hanson, L. (1991) Preparing children for hospital: a school-based intervention. In: Glasper, A. (ed.), *Child Care: Some Nursing Perspectives*. Wolfe, London, pp. 215–219.

Eland, J.M. (1985a) The role of the nurse in children's pain. In: King, K. (ed.), *Recent Advances in Nursing*. Churchill Livingstone, Edinburgh, pp. 29–45.

Eland, J.M. (1985b) The child who is hurting. *Seminars in Oncology Nursing*, **1**: 116–122.

Eland, J.M. (1988) Pharmacologic management of acute and chronic pediatric pain. *Issues in Comprehensive Pediatric Nursing*, **11**: 93–111.

Eland, J.M. and Anderson, J.E. (1977) The experience of pain in children. In: Jacox, A.

(ed.), *Pain: A Source Book for Nurses and Other Health Professionals*. Little, Brown & Co., Boston, pp. 453–473.

Elander, G., Lindberg, T. and Quarnstrom, B. (1991) Pain relief in infants after major surgery: a descriptive study. *Journal of Pediatric Surgery*, **26**(2): 128–131.

Fitzgerald, M. (1985) The postnatal department of cutaneous afferent fibre input and receptive field organization in the rat dorsal horn. *Journal of Physiology*, **364**: 1–18.

Fitzgerald, M. (1991) Development of pain mechanisms. In: Wells, J.C.D. and Woolf, C.J. (eds), *Pain Mechanisms and Management. British Medical Bulletin*, **47**(3): 667–675.

Fitzgerald, M., Millard, C. and McIntosh, N. (1989) Cutaneous sensitivity following peripheral tissue damage in newborn infants and its reversal with topical anaesthesia. *Pain*, **39**: 31–36.

Fradd, E. (1986) Learning about hospital. *Nursing Times*, **82**(3): 28–30.

Franck, L.S. (1986) A new method to quantitatively describe pain behavior in infants. *Nursing Research*, **35**(1): 28–31.

Franck, L.S. and Gregory, G.A. (1993) Clinical evaluation and treatment of infant pain in the neonatal intensive care unit. In: Schechter, N.L., Berde, C.B. and Yaster, M. (eds), *Pain in Infants, Children, and Adolescents*. Williams & Wilkins, Baltimore, pp. 519–535.

Gadish, H.S., Gonzalez, J.L. and Hayes, J.S. (1988) Factors affecting nurses' decisions to administer pediatric pain medication postoperatively. *Journal of Pediatric Nursing*, **3**(6): 383–390.

Gill, K.M., Williams, D.A., Thompson, R.J. and Kinney, T.R. (1991) Sickle cell disease in children and adolescents: the relation of child and parent pain coping strategies to adjustment. *Journal of Pediatric Psychology*, **16**(5): 643–663.

Gillies, M.J. (1993) Post operative pain in children: a review of the literature. *Journal of Clinical Nursing*, **2**: 5–10.

Glasper, A. (1991) Parents in the anaesthetic room: a blessing or a curse? In: Glasper, A. (ed.), *Child Care: Some Nursing Perspectives*. Wolfe Publishing, London, pp. 238–243.

Glasper, E.A. and Dewar, A. (1986) The results of a postal questionnaire appertaining to parental presence at the induction of anaesthesia. Unpublished. Cited in Glasper, A. (ed.), *Child Care: Some Nursing Perspectives*. Wolfe, London, pp. 238–249.

Goldman, A. and Bowman, A.(1990) The role of controlled-release morphine for pain relief in children with cancer. *Palliative Medicine*, **4**: 279–285.

Goldman, A. and Lloyd-Thomas, A.R. (1991) Pain management in children. In: Wells, J.C.D. and Woolf, C.J. (eds), *Pain Mechanisms and Management. British Medical Bulletin*, **47**(3): 676–689.

Goldman, A., Beardsmore, S. and Hunt, J. (1990) Palliative care for children with cancer: home, hospital or hospice. *Archives of Disease in Childhood*, **65**: 641–643.

Goldman, A., Feret, J., Bartolotta, C. and Weisman, S.J. (1993) Pain in terminal illness (home care). In: Schechter, N.L., Berde, C.B. and Yaster, M. (eds), *Pain in Infants, Children, and Adolescents*. Williams & Wilkins, Baltimore, pp. 425–433.

Grunau, R.V.E. and Craig, K.D. (1987) Pain expression in neonates: facial action and cry. *Pain*, **28**(3): 395–410.

Grunau, R.V.E. and Craig, K.D. (1990) Facial activity as a measure of neonatal pain expression. In: Tyler, D.C. and Krane, D.J. (eds), *Advances in Pain Research and Therapy*, Vol. 15, *Pediatric Pain*. Raven Press, New York.

Grunau, R.V.E., Johnston, C.C. and Craig, K.D. (1990) Neonatal facial and cry responses to invasive and non-invasive procedures. *Pain*, **42**: 293–305.

Gunnar, M.R., Fisch, R.O., Korsvik, S. and Donhowe, J.M. (1981) The effects of circumcision on serum cortisol and behavior. *Psychoneuroendocrinology*, **6**: 269–275.

Gunnar, M.R., Fisch, R.O. and Malone, S. (1984) The effects of pacifying stimuli in behavioral and adrenocortical responses to circumcision. *Journal of the American Academy of Child Psychiatry*, **23**: 34.

Hanallah, R.S. *et al.* (1983) Experience with parents' presence during anesthesia induction in children. *Canadian Anesthesia Society Journal*, **30**(3): 386–389.

Harmer, M. (1993) Physiology of pain and pharmacology of pain relief. In: Shankleman, J. and May, A. (eds) *Pain in Sickle Cell Disease: Setting Standards of Care*. Cardiff Sickle Cell and Thalassaemia Centre, Cardiff, pp. 21–28.

Harrison, A. (1991) Preparing children for venous blood sampling. *Pain*, **43**(3): 299–306.

Harpin, V.A. and Rutter, N. (1982) Development of emotional sweating in the newborn infant. *Archives of Disease in Childhood*, **57**: 691.

Hertzke, R.E., Fisher, D.M., Gauntlett, I.S. and Spellman, M. (1984) Are infants sensitive to respiratory depression from fentanyl? *Anesthesiology*, **67**: A512.

Hilgard, J.R. and LeBaron, S. (1984) *Hypnotherapy of Pain in Children with Cancer*. William Kauffman, Los Altos CA.

Hockenberry, M.J. (1988) Relaxation techniques in children with cancer: the nurse's role. *Journal of Association of Oncology Nursing*, **5**(1.2): 7–11.

Hockenberry, M.J. and Coody, D.K. (1986) *Pediatric Oncology and Hematology Perspectives on Care*. Mosby, St Louis, pp. 394–406.

Hodges, K., Kline, J.J., Barbero, G. and Flanery, R. (1985) Depressive symptoms in children with recurrent abdominal pain and their families. *Journal of Pediatrics*, **107**: 622–626.

Holbrook, C.T. (1990) Patient-controlled analgesia pain management for children with sickle cell disease. *Journal of Association Acad. Min. Phys.*, **1**: 93–96.

Izard, C.E. (1971) *The Face of Emotion*. Appleton-Century-Crofts, New York.

Jay, S., Ozolins, M., Elliott, C. and Caldwell, S. (1983) Assessment of children's distress during painful medical procedures. *Health Psychology*, **2**(2): 133–147.

Jay, S.M., Elliott, C.H., Katz, E.R. and Siegel, S.E. (1987) Cognitive–behavioral interventions and pharmacological interventions for children undergoing painful medical procedures. *Journal of Consulting and Clinical Psychology*, **55**: 860–865.

Johnston, C.C., Stevens, B., Craig, K.D. and Grunau, R.V.E. (1993) Developmental changes in pain expression in premature, full-term, two- and four-month-old infants. *Pain*, **52**: 201–208.

Klein, E.R.(1992) Premedicating children for painful invasive procedures. *Journal of Pediatric Oncology Nursing*, **9**(4): 170–179.

Koren, G., Butt, W., Chinyanga, H., Soldin, S., Tan, Y-K. and Pape, K. (1985) Postoperative morphine infusion in newborn infants: assessment of disposition characteristics and safety. *Journal of Pediatrics*, **107**(6): 963–967.

Lander, J., Fowler-Kerry, S. and Oberle, S. (1982) Children's venepuncture pain: influence of technical factors. *Journal of Pain and Symptom Management*, **7**(6): 343–349.

Langworthy, O.R. (1933) Development of behavior patterns and myelinization of the nervous system in the human fetus and infant. *Carnegie Contributions to Embryology*, **24**: 3.

Levine, J.D. and Gordon, N.C. (1982) Pain in prelingual children and its evaluation by pain-induced vocalization. *Pain*, **14**: 85–93.

Ludwig, M.A. and Beam, T. (1992) Alterations in immune system function. In: Castiglia, P.T. and Harbin, R.C. (eds) *Child Health Care: Process and Practice*. Lippincott, Philadelphia.

Månsson E.M., Bjørkhem, G. and Wiebe, T. (1993) The effect of preparation for lumbar puncture on children undergoing chemotherapy. *Oncology Nursing Forum*, **20**(1): 39–45.

Marchette, L., Main, T.R., Redick, E., Bagg, A. and Leatherland, J. (1991) Pain reduction interventions during neonatal circumcision. *Nursing Research*, **40**(4): 241–244.

Marks, K. (1992) Children's pain after operations 'often undertreated'., *The Independent*, 2 June.

Mather, L. and Mackie, J. (1983) The incidence of post-operative pain in children. *Pain*, **15**: 271–282.

Mathews, J.R., McGrath, P.J. and Pigeon, H. (1993) Assessment and measurement of pain in children. In: Schechter, N.L., Berde, C.B. and Yaster, M.(eds), *Pain in Infants, Children, and Adolescents*. Williams & Wilkins, Baltimore, pp. 97–111.

McCaffery, M. and Beebe, A. (1989) *Pain: Clinical Manual for Nursing Practice*. Mosby, St Louis.

McGrath, P.A. (1990) *Pain in Children: Nature, Assessment, and Treatment*. Guilford Press, New York.

McGrath, P. and de Veber, L.L. (1986) The management of acute pain evoked by medical procedures in children with cancer. *Journal of Pain and Symptom Management*, **1**(3): 145–150.

McGrath, P.J. and Unruh, A. (1987) *Pain in Children and Adolescents*. Elsevier, Amsterdam.

McGraw, M.B. (1941) Neural mechanisms as exemplified by changing reactions of the infant to pinprick. *Child Development*, **12**: 31–41.

McIlvaine, W.B. (1989) Perioperative pain management in children: a review. *Journal of Pain and Symptom Management*, **4**(4): 215–229.

McIntosh, N., van Veen, L. and Brameyer, H. (1993) The pain of heel prick and its measurement in preterm infants. *Pain*, **52**: 71–74.

McLauglin, C.R., Hull, J.G., Edwards, W.H., Cramer, C.P. and Dewey, W.L. (1993) Neonatal pain: a comprehensive survey of attitudes and practices. *Journal of Pain and Symptom Management*, **8**(1): 7–16.

Melamed, B.G. and Siegel, L.J. (1975) Reduction of anxiety in children facing hospitalization and surgery by use of filmed modelling. *Journal of Consultant Clinical Psychology*, **43**: 511–521.

Melamed, B.G., Dearborn, M. and Hermecz, D.A. (1983) Necessary considerations for surgery preparation: age and previous experience. *Psychosomatic Medicine*, **45**: 517–525.

Merskey, H. and Spear, F.G. (1967) *Pain: Psychological and Psychiatric Aspects*. Baillière Tindall & Cassell, London.

Miser, A.W. (1993) Management of pain associated with childhood cancer. In: Schechter, N.L., Berde, C.B., and Yaster, M. (eds), *Pain in Infants, Children, and Adolescents*. Williams & Wilkins, Baltimore, pp. 411–423.

Miser, A.W., Miser, J.S. and Clarke, B.S. (1980) Continuous intravenous infusion of morphine sulphate for control of severe pain in children with terminal malignancy. *Journal of Pediatrics*, **96**; 930–932.

Miser, A.W., McCalla, J., Dothage, J.A., Wesley, M. and Miser, J.S. (1987a) Pain as a presenting symptom in children and young adults with newly diagnosed malignancy. *Pain*, **29**: 85–90.

Miser, A.W., Dothage, J.A., Wesley, R.A. and Miser, J.S. (1987b) The prevalence of pain in a pediatric and young adult cancer population. *Pain*, **29**: 73–83.

Morrison, R.A. and Vedro, D.A. (1989) Pain management in the child with sickle cell disease. *Pediatric Nursing*, **15**(6): 595–599, 613.

Myron, A.V. and Maguire, D.P. (1991) Pain perception in the neonate: implications for circumcision. *Journal of Professional Nursing*, **7**(3): 188–195.

Newburger, P.E. and Sallan, S.E. (1981) Chronic pain: principles of management. *Journal of Pediatrics*, **98**: 180–189.

Olness, K. (1981) Imagery (self-hypnosis) as adjunct therapy in childhood cancer: clinical experience with 25 patients. *American Journal of Pediatric Hematology and Oncology*, **3**: 313–321.

O'Malley, M.E. and McNamara, S.T. (1993) Children's drawing: preoperative assessment tool. *AORN Journal*, **57**(5): 1074–1089.

Orlowski, J.P. (1986) Cerebrospinal fluid endorphins and the infant apnoea syndrome. *Pediatrics*, **78**: 233–237.

Owens, M.E. (1984) Pain in infancy: conceptual and methodological issues. *Pain*, **20**: 213–230.

Owens, M.E. and Todt, E.H. (1984) Pain in infancy: neonatal reaction to a heel lance. *Pain*, **20**: 77–86.

Page, G.G. (1991) Chronic pain and the child with juvenile rheumatoid arthritis. *Journal of Pediatric Health Care*, **5**(1): 18–23.

Page-Goertz, S.S. (1989) Even children have arthritis. *Pediatric Nursing*, **15**(1): 11–16.

Patterson, K.L. and Lewis Ware, L. (1988) Coping skills for children undergoing painful medical procedures. *Issues in Comprehensive Pediatric Nursing*, **11**: 113–143.

Pegelow, C.H. (1992) Survey of pain management therapy provided for children with sickle cell disease. *Clinical Pediatrics*, **31**(4): 211–214.

Porter, F. (1989) Pain in the Newborn. *Clinics in Perinatology*, **16**(2): 549–564.

Purcell-Jones, G., Dormon, F. and Summer, E. (1987) The use of opioids in neonates: a retrospective study of 933 cases. *Anaesthesia*, **42**: 1316–1320.

Purcell-Jones, G., Dormon, F. and Summer, E. (1988) Pediatric anaesthetists' perceptions of neonatal and infant pain. *Pain*, **33**: 181–188.

Rawlings, D.J., Miller, P.A. and Engel, R.R. (1980) The effect of circumcision on transcutaneous pO_2 in term infants. *American Journal of Disease in Childhood*, **13**: 676.

Rivera, W.B. (1991) Practical points in the assessment and management of postoperative pediatric pain. *Journal of Post Anesthetic Nursing*, **6**(1): 40–42.

Roop Moyer, S.M. and Howe, C.J. (1991) Pediatric pain intervention in the PACU. *Critical Care Nursing Clinics of North America*, **3**(1): 49–57.

Ross, D.M. and Ross, S.A. (1988) Assessment of pediatric pain: an overview. *Issues in Comprehensive Pediatric Nursing*, **11**: 73–91.

Sartori, P.C.E., Gordon, P.G.J. and Darbyshire, P.J. (1990) Continuous papaveretum infusion for the control of pain in painful sickling crisis. *Archives of Disease in Childhood*, March: 1151–1153.

Schechter, N., Allan, D.A. and Hanson, K. (1986) Status of pediatric pain control: a comparison of hospital usage in children and adults. *Pediatrics*, **77**(1): 11–15.

Schechter, N.L., Berrian, F.B. and Katz, S.M. (1988) The use of patient-controlled analgesia in adolescents with sickle cell pain crisis: a preliminary report. *Journal of Pain and Symptom Management*, **3**: 109–113.

Shankleman, J. and May, A. (1993) *Pain in Sickle Cell Disease: Setting Standards of Care*. Cardiff Sickle Cell and Thalassaemia Centre, Cardiff.

Shapiro, B. (1993) Management of painful episodes in Sickle Cell Disease. In: Schechter, N.L., Berde, C.B. and Yaster, M. (eds), *Pain in Infants, Children, and Adolescents*. Williams & Wilkins, Baltimore, pp. 385–410.

Shapiro, B.S., Dinges, D.F., Carota Orne, E., Ohene-Frempong, K. and Orne, M.T. (1990) Recording of crisis pain in sickle cell disease. In: Tyler, D.C. and Krane, E.J. (eds), *Advances in Pain Research Therapy*, Vol. 15. Raven Press, New York, pp. 313–321.

Shelley, P. (1993) Giving children a voice: a profile of Action for Sick Children. *Child Health*, **1**(1): 21–24.

Southall, D.P., Cronin, B.C., Hartmann, H., Harrison-Sewell, C. and Samuels, M.P. (1993) Invasive procedures in children receiving intensive care. *British Medical Journal*, **306**: 1512–1513.

Spitzer, A. (1993) The significance of pain in children's experiences of hemophilia. *Clinical Nursing Research*, **2**(1): 5–18.

Sutters, K.A. and Miaskowski, C. (1992) The problem of pain in children with cancer: a research review. *Oncology Nursing Forum*, **19**(3): 465–471.

Swafford, L.I. and Allen, D. (1968) Pain relief in the pediatric patient. *Medical Clinics of North America*, **52**(1): 131–136.

Thompson, K.L., Varni, J.W. and Hanson, V. (1987) Comprehensive assessment of pain in juvenile rheumatoid arthritis: an empirical model. *Journal of Pediatric Psychology*, **12**: 241–255.

Tong, R., Shimomura, S. and Rotblatt, M. (1980) Meperidine-induced seizures in sickle cell patients. *Hospital Formulary*, **76**: 764–772.

Torres, F. and Anderson, C. (1985) The normal EEG of the human newborn. *Journal of Clinical Neurophysiology*, **2**: 89–103.

Vandenberg, K.A. and Franck, L.S. (1990) Behavioral issues for infants with BPD. In: Lund, C.H. (ed.) *Bronchopulmonary Dysplasia: Strategies for Total Patient*

Care. Neonatal Network, Petalume, CA.

Varni, J.W. and Walco, G.A. (1988) Chronic and recurrent pain associated with pediatric chronic diseases. *Issues in Comprehensive Pediatric Nursing*, **11**: 145–158.

Visintainer, M.A. and Wolfer, J.A. (1975) Psychological preparation for surgical pediatric patients: the effect on children's and parents' stress responses and adjustment. *Pediatrics*, **56**: 187–202.

Volpe, J. (1981) *Neurology of the Newborn*. Saunders, Philadelphia.

Walco, G.A. and Oberlander, T.F. (1993) Musculoskeletal pain syndromes in children. In: Schechter, N.L., Berde, C.B. and Yaster, M. (eds), *Pain in Infants, Children, and Adolescents*. Williams & Wilkins, Baltimore, pp. 459–471.

Walco, G.A., Dampier, C.D., Hartstein, G., Djordjevic, D. and Miller, L. (1990) The relationship between recurrent clinical pain and pain threshold in children. In: Tyler, D.C. and Krane, E.J. (eds), *Advances in Pain Research and Therapy*, Vol. 15. Raven Press, New York. pp. 333–340.

Wark, K.J. (1991) Pediatric anesthesia. In: Adams, A.P. and Cashman, J.N. (eds), *Anaesthesia, Analgesia and Intensive Care*. Edward Arnold, London, pp. 189–209.

Webster, D.E. (1993) Chronic and recurrent pain during childhood. In: Ramamurthy, S. and Roger, J.N. (eds), *Decision Making in Pain Management*. Mosby-Year Book, St Louis, pp. 162–165.

Williams, J. (1987) Managing paediatric pain. *Nursing Times*, **83**:36–39.

Williamson, P.S. and Williamson, R.N. (1983) Physiologic stress reduction by local anesthetic during newborn circumcision. *Pediatrics*, **71**: 36–40.

Wolff, P.H. (1969) The natural history of crying and other vocalizations in early infancy. In: Foss, B. (ed) *Determinants of Infant Behaviour*, vol. 4. Methuen, London, pp. 81–115.

Wolff, P.H. (1974) Active language: the natural history of crying and other vocalizations in early infancy. In: Stone, L.J., Smith, H.T. and Murphy, L.B. (eds) *The Competent Infant*. Tavistock Publications, London.

Yaster, M. (1987) Analgesia and anesthesia in neonates. *Journal of Pediatrics*, **111**: 394–395.

Zelter, L. and LeBaron, S. (1982) Hypnosis and nonhypnotic teaching for reduction of pain and anxiety during painful procedures in children and adolescents with cancer. *Journal of Pediatrics*, **101**: 1032–1035.

Zelter, L. and LeBaron, S. (1986) The hypnotic treatment of children in pain. In: Wolraich, M. and Routh, D.K. (eds), *Advances in Developmental and Behavioral Pediatrics*. JAI Press, Greenwich, pp. 197–234.

Children's pain: the future   7

Attitudes, understanding, knowledge, research and practice have come a long way since the 1970s when children's pain was tentatively established as an issue worthy of real consideration. The body of knowledge which is available is growing in both breadth and depth and is now much more representative of the multidimensional nature of pain. Scientists, clinicians, psychologists, philosophers, pharmacologists, surgeons, anaesthetists, nurses and above all the children and their families have all contributed to the understanding of the complex issues surrounding management of children's pain. Each discipline has added a new perspective to understanding. However, despite all of the above knowledge some children continue to suffer pain. It is well established that theory alone is not the answer to the practical problem of managing a child's pain – the theory has to be implemented wherever and whenever children are liable to find themselves in a painful situation. The transition from theory to practice is fundamental – every nurse who cares for children has a responsibility to develop their knowledge and skills in respect to pain prevention and pain management. The theory that has been developed must be critically considered and then, as appropriate, implemented in practice – the separation of theory and practice that is evident in many areas of nursing must be bridged if care is to develop (Kim, 1993). Theory must challenge practice and, as importantly, practice must challenge theory. Every nurse must question themselves as to how they as an individual and as a member of a multidisciplinary team can contribute to reducing a child's pain.

Pain management is ultimately one of the most rewarding aspects to nursing care both on a professional and on a personal level. Nurses are there to care for the child and their family. Fulfilling the child's basic need and right to be pain free is a fundamental aspect of the caring role. Nursing care that does not acknowledge pain management as a priority cannot legitimately be seen to be care. The nurturing component of nursing requires anxiety and pain to be considered. The domain of nursing requires the child to be the central focus of care and if nurses are truly assessing *the child's needs* then pain would clearly be established as a priority need and a therapeutic relationship can be established (Kitson, 1993; Leininger, 1978; Watson, 1985).

Nurses require to be fully informed about the latest research findings and developments/innovations in practice. Nurse specialists and members of pain management teams can be a crucial part of the facilitation of nursing development. The role of both must initially be to serve the best interest of the child but this may be fulfilled in many ways. One way is by networking with all the practitioners involved in caring for the child so that they are kept informed of developments in care and practice. The role of the specialist nurse should not be to deskill their colleagues by becoming the sole resource and 'the expert' within the community or hospital setting. The aim should be to promote and facilitate evolution (and perhaps even revolution) within and by colleagues. Specialized pain management courses devoted to the specific needs and challenges of caring for children of whatever age need to be, and are being, developed. These courses should provide a foundation for the development of enhanced levels of practice.

Further research is required, especially research based within the British health care arena, since the majority of research has been undertaken within the USA. Obviously much of this has relevance to British children, their needs and to the professionals caring for them. However, considering the impact that societal, cultural and contextual factors have on the child's experience of pain, further investigation is crucial within British practice settings. It would be interesting, for example, to determine whether the word lists developed in the USA have relevance within Britain and whether or not they have relevance within the different regions of the British Isles. Some of the established pain tools still require further research to strengthen them as tools and to establish their credibility within a wide range of pain situations. The need for the development of a neonatal pain assessment tool is clearly established and this must be met in the near future.

Copp (1990) identifies a range of domains of inquiry which she sees as highlighting areas in which research has been carried out. She suggests that despite the unevenness with which some of these areas have been studied nurse researchers should consider all areas as important (Table 7.1). Every single one of Copp's domains is under-researched within the speciality of children's pain and each and every one needs to be addressed as a matter of urgency. Without information and knowledge of all these areas the developing body of knowledge in respect to children's pain is incomplete.

Additionally children deserve a service of the highest quality and part of the process in developing such a service lies in the development of standards of care. These standards of care must be developed by the multidisciplinary team in consultation with children and their families. Moves to standard

Table 7.1 Copp domains of inquiry in pain research
(Copp, 1990)

Pain assessment
Pain and suffering as human response
Pain and organ specificity
Pain and disease specificity
Pain and body system specificity
Pain measurement tools
Pain and time
Non-pharmacological intervention modalities
Pain and care setting
Pain in those populations at risk
Pain responses culturally expressed
Iatrogenic pain
Pain advocacy and social action
Pain and education
Multidisciplinary approaches to pain
Causes and theories of pain
Pharmacological intervention modalities
Epidemiology of pain
Pain, values and ethics
Pain prevention
Quality assessment and pain management
Pain policy
Pain politics and economics
Pain caused by environment and natural catastrophe
Pain caused by man-made error/intention

---

setting must be seen to be a priority if the performance of pain management services is to be measured (Fig. 7.1). Obviously, owing to the
highly individualized nature of pain, standard setting can be problematic
but this should not prevent standards from being formulated. Øvretveit
(1992) sees standard setting and quality as a means of continuously improving services.

Quality assurance and quality audit in respect to pain management
are vital components of a developing service. A quality pain service
requires to be integrated, systematic and comprehensive and it is as important for the members of the multidisciplinary team to be involved in
a quality-driven and innovative service as it is for the children and their
families.

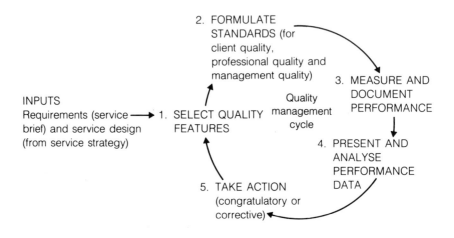

Figure 7.1 The quality management cycle. (Reproduced with permission from Øvretveit, *Health Service Quality: An Introduction to Quality Methods for Health Services*; published by Blackwell Scientific Publications, 1992)

REFERENCES

Copp, L.A. (1990) The patient in pain: USA nursing research. In: Bergman, R. (ed.), *Nursing Research for Nursing Practice: An International Perspective*. Chapman & Hall, London, pp. 124–144.

Kim, H.S. (1993) Putting theory into practice: problems and prospects. *Journal of Advanced Nursing*, **18**: 1632–1639.

Kitson, A. (1993) Formalising concepts related to nursing and caring. In: Kitson, A. (ed.), *Nursing: Art and Science*. Chapman & Hall, London, pp. 25–47.

Leninger, M. (1978) *Transcultural Nursing: Concepts, Theories and Practices*. Wiley, New York.

Øvretveit, J. (1992) *Health Service Quality: An Introduction to Quality Methods for Health Services*. Blackwell Scientific Publications, Oxford.

Watson, J. (1985) *Nursing: Human Science and Human Care*. Appleton-Century-Crofts, Newark, CT.

Index

By the same author
Manual of Paediatric Intensive Care Nursing

Edited by **B Carter,** Department of Health Care Studies,
Manchester Metropolitan University, UK

'Well laid out and user friendly, with a wide selection of
references on each area covered...This publication is the result
of the collaboration of various paediatric intensive care
specialists which, in a predominantly American field, makes
a refreshing change'
- Nursing Times

The first British publication of its kind, the *Manual of Paediatric Intensive
Care Nursing* provides clear, concise guidance that will be of benefit to
both practising and student ICU nurses alike. Key symptoms and
conditions such as pain, respiratory disorders and cardiovascular
problems are comprehensively dealt with in separate chapters, and there
is also a section on nursing critically ill neonates.

» first British paediatric intensive care manual for nurses

» considers the physical, psycho-social and spiritual need of children in
intensive care

» adopts an holistic approach

» explores the nursing care required by children with a variety of needs
and problems e.g. the child in pain, the child with respiratory
problems, care of the neonate

Contents: The ethos of paediatric intensive care. Care of the child with
compromised immunology and infection. Care of the neonate. Care of the
child with respiratory problems. Care of the child with cardiovascular
problems. Care of the child with neurological needs. Care of the child with
acute renal failure. Care of the child with polytrauma and thermal injury.
Care of the child in pain. Care of the dying child. The ongoing care of the
child. Paediatric pharmacology. Appendix. Support Groups. Index.

c.368pp: 234x156: 30 line drawings: 1993 Paperback: 0-412-44050-4: £19.99

CHAPMAN & HALL

Lippincott Manual of Paediatric Nursing

3rd edition

L S Brunner, Consultant in Nursing, Yale University School of Nursing, USA and
D S Suddarth, Consultant in Health Occupations, Alexandria Hospital School of Nursing, USA

Adapted for the UK by **Barbara F Weller**

'an excellent source of references' - Nursing Standard

This new edition provides complete coverage for the care of the unwell child. It retains many of the features from previous editions which readers have found useful and also incorporates a great deal of new material. An individualized approach to care is given throughout and a guide is included for assessing the child's and the family's needs with the identification of potential problems. In describing clinical procedures, care has been taken to adhere to principles and nursing research when giving a rationale for action.

» care structured around stages of the nursing process

» list format for quick reference

» parental participation and family-centred care emphasized

Contents: Preface. Child health maintenance. The sick child. Paediatric clinical nursing practice. Problems of infants. Care of the child with a respiratory disorder. Care of the child with a cardiovascular disorder. Care of the child with a blood disorder. Care of the child with a gastrointestinal disorder. Care of the child with a metabolic or endocrine disorder. Care of the child with a renal or genitourinary disorder. Care of the child with an orthopaedic disorder. Care of the child with a connective tissue disorder. Care of the child with an eye, ear or nose and throat disorder. Care of the child with a neurological disorder. Care of the child with cancer. The child with special needs. Special paediatric problems. Index.

624pp: 246x189: Illus: 1991 Hardback: 0-412-53180-1: £16.99

CHAPMAN & HALL

Neonatal Nursing

D A Crawford, Neonatal Nursing Unit, Leicester Royal Infirmary, UK and **M Morris,** formerly of Neonatal Nursing Unit, Leicester Royal Infirmary, UK

Neonatal Nursing offers a systematic approach to the nursing care of the sick newborn baby. Nursing actions and responsibilities are the focus of the text with relevant research findings, clinical applications, anatomy, physiology and pathology provided where necessary. This comprehensive text covers all areas of neonatal nursing including ethics, continuing care in the community, intranatal care, statistics and pharmokinetics so that holistic care of the infant is described.

» first British book on neonatal nursing, written by nurses for nurses, it is a comprehensive text covering all aspects of the neonatal nursing unit

» the book is written using explained terminology and a wealth of references so that it will be invaluable to both neonatal nurses, paediatric nurses, midwives and their students to help them understand the basic concepts of neonatal nursing and expand their knowledge further

Contents: Preface. Neonatal care today. Nursing models - a suitable framework for care? Prenatal and intranatal care of the foetus, mother and father. Resuscitation - flying squad transfer. Nursing care of babies who are born too soon or too small. Nursing care of a baby with a disorder of the gastrointestinal system. Feeding low birthweight infants in today's neonatal environment. Nursing care of a baby with a disorder of the respiratory system. Nursing care of a baby with a disorder of the cardiovascular system. Nursing care of a baby with a disorder of the nervous system. Nursing care of a baby in renal failure. Neonatal infection. Nursing care of a baby with jaundice. Nursing care of a baby in pain and discomfort. Enhancing development through play. Neonatal pharmacy. Ethical issues in the neonatal unit. Home oxygenation. Infant statistics. Appendix 1: Tables of normal values. Appendix 2: Assessment of gestational age. Appendix 3: List of abbreviations.

c.416pp: 234x156: 22 line illus: August 1994 Paperback: 0-412-48730-6: £16.99

CHAPMAN & HALL

Pain

A handbook for nurses

2nd edition

B Sofaer, Nursing Research Unit, University of Brighton, UK

'...a must for the learner at whatever stage.'
- *Journal of District Nursing* (review of the first edition)

'...more nurses are seeking an introduction to the subject. The new edition of this handbook could be just what they are looking for...a welcome edition to the series. Its philosophy will not date...'
- *Nursing Times*

This new edition helps nurses to understand the complex phenomenon of pain. Building upon the success of the first edition, this text introduces nurses to the physical, psychological, spiritual and cultural factors influencing pain, together with methods of pain assessment and appropriate therapies.

» considers pain from both patients' and nurses' view points

» examines the physical, psychological and cultural aspects of pain

» includes a new chapter on the role of nursing in pain management

Contents: Preface. A patient's experience. Towards an understanding of pain. The uniqueness of the individual. The unique position of the nurse. Accountability, responsibility and communication. Assessing pain. Pain therapies. Feelings about pain. The role of nursing in pain management - some thoughts for the future. Glossary. General bibliography. Index.

99pp: 216x138: Illus: July 1992, Paperback: 0-412-44010-5: £9.99

CHAPMAN & HALL